THE SOOTHING SPOON

VIRGINIA CUNNINGHAM

THE SOOTHING SPOON

Satisfying Recipes for Lifelong Wellness and Comfort

Virginia J. Cunningham

COPYRIGHT 2025

All rights reserved. No part of this publication may be reproduced, distributed, or transmitted in any form or by any means, including photocopying, recording, or other electronic or mechanical methods, without the prior written permission of the publisher, except in the case of brief quotations embodied in critical reviews and certain other noncommercial uses permitted by copyright law.

TABLE OF CONTENT

Introduction 5

1: An Anti-Inflammatory Diet, Really? 7

2: Breakfast and Brunch 14

3: Plant-Based Meals 32

4: Grains and Pasta 43

5: Salads and Light Meals 57

6: Fish and Seafoods 72

7: Slow Cooker Options 81

8: Smoothies, Teas, and Beverages 101

9: Long-Term Management Advice 112

4 weeks meal plan 114

Recipe index 117

INTRODUCTION

Inflammation, whether chronic or acute, is associated with over 50% of all fatalities on Earth. Some of the most prevalent long-term health problems, including diabetes, heart disease, autoimmune disorders, and even some cancers, have this as their underlying cause. Surprisingly, our daily decisions—including our diet, lifestyle, and stress management techniques—are actually exacerbating inflammation, even though nearly **6 in 10 adults in the United States** deal with inflammatory-related chronic conditions.

The effects of inflammation are likely familiar to you if you are reading this. Maybe it manifests as a morning ache in one or more of your joints. Even if it's just chronic gas, it can make you feel like your body is secretly fighting you. Perhaps it's an autoimmune disorder that unannounced itself and turned your world upside down. You might be experiencing the universal sensation of unease. Minimal power consumption. Cloudy thinking. Stiff, achy, tired, and unsure why.

Let me tell you something. You are not alone. And you are not imagining it. Chronic inflammation is a real, insidious problem, but there is good news: it is not a life sentence.

This book isn't about quick fixes, fad diets, or avoiding certain food groups for no reason. It is about nourishing your body so that it can fight inflammation from within. It's about realizing that food is more than just calories or fuel; it's information. Every bite you take sends a message to your body, either "heal" or "harm."

The anti-inflammatory diet is based on science, and the results speak for themselves. According to studies, eating a diet high in anti-inflammatory foods can reduce your risk of chronic disease, increase your energy, and even help you age gracefully. A landmark study published in the journal *Nature Medicine* discovered that a Mediterranean-style diet—rich in anti-inflammatory foods like olive oil, fish, and leafy greens—reduced inflammatory markers in just **8 weeks**. Imagine what could happen in eight months. Or a lifetime.

But this book isn't just about science; it's also about storytelling. It's about how real people, including myself, have applied these principles to create a lifestyle that heals, energizes, and transforms. And let me tell you, the journey was not always smooth. I've experienced my fair share of turmeric-stained countertops, failed recipes, and moments of doubt. But I've also had moments of clarity—the first time I awoke without joint pain, the day I realized I could eat a meal without bloating, and the gradual but steady realization that I was regaining control of my health.

Why You Need This Book

The truth is that inflammation is not limited to people suffering from chronic illnesses. It's a problem for everyone. Stress, poor sleep, pollution, sedentary lifestyles, and ultra-processed foods all contribute to low-grade chronic inflammation, even if the symptoms are not immediately apparent. It's like a silent fire smoldering beneath the surface, and if left unchecked, it can lead to larger problems in the future.

But here's the best part: you can extinguish the fire. This book will teach you how. You'll learn what inflammation is and how it affects your body (spoiler: it's more than just pain and swelling).
- Surprising foods and environmental triggers that could be fueling the fire.
- Delicious, nutrient-dense foods that function as fire extinguishers for your body.
- Practical advice for making lifestyle changes that last—because, let's face it, no one has time for a 10-step smoothie ritual every morning.

When I first began this journey, I was overwhelmed. I was tired of feeling bad and frustrated by all the contradictory advice out there. But, with trial and error and a lot of garlic, I eventually found my way. And now I'd like to help you find yours.

This is more than just a diet book; it's a guide to improving your relationship with your body and health. It's about regaining control. And along the way, I promise we'll laugh, learn, and maybe even spill some turmeric on the counter.

So grab a cup of green tea, settle in, and let's embark on this journey together. Because, while inflammation is powerful, with the right tools, you are as well.

1. An Anti-inflammatory Diet, Really?

Have you ever felt like your body was trying to send you a message, but you ignored it because life was just too busy? That was me before I discovered the anti-inflammatory diet. Picture this: I was sitting on my couch one evening, knees aching like I'd just climbed Mount Everest (I hadn't), my stomach in knots from yet another mystery meal that didn't agree with me, and my energy levels scraping the floor. It was then I realized—this wasn't normal. Something had to change.

The anti-inflammatory diet isn't some trendy detox where you drink kale smoothies for a week and call it a lifestyle change. No, it's a long-term approach to eating that's rooted in science, designed to heal, nourish, and protect your body from the inside out. At its core, the aim of the anti-inflammatory diet is to reduce chronic inflammation, which is often the sneaky culprit behind many modern health issues—arthritis, heart disease, diabetes, and even that stubborn fatigue that makes getting out of bed feel like running a marathon.

Why Anyone Would Need It

Have you ever felt like your body was trying to send you a message, but you ignored it because you were too busy? That was me before I learned about the anti-inflammatory diet. Picture this: I was sitting on my couch one evening, knees aching like I'd just climbed Mount Everest (I hadn't), stomach in knots from yet another mystery meal that didn't agree with me, and energy levels dropping to the floor. It was then that I realized something wasn't right. Something needed to change.

The anti-inflammatory diet is not some trendy detox in which you drink kale smoothies for a week and claim to have changed your lifestyle. No, it's a long-term, scientifically based eating plan designed to heal, nourish, and protect your body from within. The anti-inflammatory diet's primary goal is to reduce chronic inflammation, which is frequently the hidden cause of many modern health problems—arthritis, heart disease, diabetes, and even stubborn fatigue that makes getting out of bed feel like a marathon.

Why Does Anyone Need It?

Let us talk about inflammation. In moderation, it can be beneficial. When you scrape your knee, your body responds with redness, swelling, and heat to repair the damage. That's acute inflammation, and your body is responding like a well-trained firefighter. But what happens if the fire never goes out? Chronic inflammation is like a low-level fire burning inside you, caused by a poor diet, stress, a lack of sleep, and other modern-day triggers. It has a negative impact on your health over time, contributing to autoimmune diseases and mental fog.

So, why should someone follow an anti-inflammatory diet? Because it's like pressing the reset button. It helps to calm the internal fire and provides your body with the resources it requires to function optimally. This diet is a game changer if you have an autoimmune condition, are struggling with weight gain, or simply want to feel more like yourself again. And, believe me, it's not about deprivation; it's about learning to love food that loves you back.

Who Could Benefit from It

What is the short answer? Nearly everyone. Here's why: chronic inflammation does not discriminate. It infiltrates the lives of the young and old, athletes and couch potatoes alike. However, some people will benefit more significantly from adopting an anti-inflammatory lifestyle.

- Those with Chronic Conditions: If you have rheumatoid arthritis, lupus, fibromyalgia, or another inflammatory condition, this diet could change your life.
- People Struggling with Gut Issues: Bloating, gas, IBS, and food sensitivities are common indicators that your gut needs some TLC—and an anti-inflammatory diet is a great place to start.
- The Chronically Tired: If your "tired" is tired, inflammation could be the cause. This diet can help to maintain energy levels.
- Anyone Overwhelmed by Stress: Stress causes inflammation, and eating anti-inflammatory foods can help to reduce the damage.
- People Who Want to Age Gracefully: Chronic inflammation hastens aging. An anti-inflammatory diet can help you stay active and healthy for years to come.

How to Benefit From It

Here is where things become practical. Knowing that an anti-inflammatory diet is beneficial is one thing; however, how do you put it into practice in your daily life?

- ❖ Begin Small: Don't completely overhaul your pantry overnight (unless you're feeling especially brave). Start by including more anti-inflammatory foods in your diet, such as leafy greens, berries, and fatty fish.
- ❖ Ditch the Inflammatory Villains: Eliminate processed foods, sugary drinks, and refined carbohydrates. Yes, I understand that last one hurts—but you'll thank me later.
- ❖ Experiment with Spices: Turmeric, ginger, and cinnamon aren't just for Instagrammable lattes. They are inflammation-fighting superheroes who can enhance the flavor of your meals.
- ❖ Listen to Your Body: Every journey is unique. Pay attention to how different foods make you feel, and make adjustments accordingly.
- ❖ Make it Fun: Find recipes that you enjoy, involve your family, and celebrate small victories. The goal is to establish a lifestyle, not a punishment.

When I first decided to try an anti-inflammatory diet, I didn't intend to write a book or become a wellness expert. Honestly, all I wanted was to feel better. I wanted to wake up without joint pain, eat without regret, and have enough energy to get through the day without crashing.

At first, I assumed it would be a chore. I imagined long grocery lists, bland meals, and numerous sacrifices. But what I discovered was the exact opposite. This journey turned out to be one of discovery—learning new recipes, trying new ingredients, and, most importantly, understanding my body in ways I hadn't before.

Anti-inflammatory Powerhouses

Allow me to introduce you to the VIPs of the anti-inflammatory world—the powerhouses. These foods are like nutrition's Avengers, swooping in to combat inflammation and save the day. They're high in nutrients, antioxidants, and compounds that help your body regulate its internal processes. But don't be intimidated by their superfood status. They're not here to pass judgment on your previous experiences with instant noodles or late-night pizza binges (trust me, I've been there).

When I first heard about these "powerhouses," I expected them to be exotic, expensive, and difficult to pronounce. Spoiler alert: they are not. In fact, many of them had been quietly sitting in my pantry all along, waiting for me to unlock their full potential. The first time I purchased turmeric, I thought, "Great, now I just need to figure out what to do with this orange powder." Little did I know it would quickly become my secret weapon.

1. Turmeric, the Golden Wonder

Turmeric is like that friend who excels at everything but remains humble about it. It contains curcumin, a compound that has strong anti-inflammatory and antioxidant properties. Including a pinch of turmeric in your meals is like giving your body a warm, healing hug.

The first time I used turmeric, I became overly ambitious. I decided to make a golden milk latte, envisioning a warm, Instagrammable masterpiece. Instead, I got a lumpy, mustard-yellow concoction that tasted like I had accidentally spilled curry powder in my coffee. My kitchen resembled a crime scene, and my blender still has turmeric stains to this day. Lesson learned: begin small and blend thoroughly.

Now, I sprinkle turmeric on roasted vegetables, soups, and even scrambled eggs. Pro tip: pair it with black pepper to increase absorption.

2. Berries: Tiny But Mighty

Blueberries, strawberries, and raspberries are packed with antioxidants and vitamins. They are nature's candy, without the sugar crash. Berries are particularly high in anthocyanins, which help to reduce inflammation and protect cells from damage.

My first "berry binge" is still vivid in my memory. I purchased a large container of blueberries and decided to eat them straight from the tub while binge-watching a crime drama. Everything was going well until I accidentally knocked over the tub, spilling blueberries all over my couch. It resembled a blueberry massacre. On the bright side, my dog was ecstatic.

Nowadays, I'm a little more civilized about my berry consumption. I add them to smoothies, sprinkle them on oatmeal, or simply snack on them (carefully) throughout the day.

3. Leafy Greens

Leafy greens such as spinach, kale, and Swiss chard are like dependable supporting characters in a film. They may not steal the show, but without them, the plot crumbles. These greens are anti-inflammatory gold, rich in vitamins, minerals, and fiber.

When I first tried kale, I wasn't particularly impressed. Raw, it tasted like punishment. But then I discovered the wonders of kale chips. One Sunday, I tossed some kale leaves in olive oil, sprinkled with sea salt, and baked. I felt like a culinary genius—until I got distracted scrolling through my phone and burned the entire batch. For hours, my kitchen smelled of charred disappointment.

Now I've mastered the art of kale. To soften the leaves for salads, I massage them with a little olive oil and lemon juice. I also add it to soups and stir-fries for a quick nutritional boost.

4. Salmon, the Omega-3 King

Fatty fish, such as salmon, contain omega-3 fatty acids, which act as anti-inflammatory firefighters. They help to extinguish the flames of chronic inflammation and keep your heart and brain healthy.

The first time I cooked salmon, I almost triggered the smoke alarm. I had no idea what I was doing and overcooked it until it was dry enough to be used as a doorstop. But, hey, we can learn from our mistakes, right?

Now, salmon is one of my favorite meals. I bake it with a simple honey-mustard glaze or grill it with a lemon squeeze. It's tasty, simple, and makes me feel fancy—even if I'm eating it in my pajamas.

5. Avocado

Avocado is the darling of the wellness world, and with good reason. It's rich in healthy fats, fiber, and anti-inflammatory compounds. It also tastes great on almost anything.

My first avocado toast experience was underwhelming. I spread the avocado too thickly and used way too much salt. It felt like licking a salt lick. But once I figured out the proper balance, I was hooked. I now use avocado in smoothies, salads, and even as a substitute for butter in baking.

6. Nuts and Seeds

Almonds, walnuts, chia seeds, and flaxseeds are small but powerful superfoods. They contain healthy fats, fiber, and anti-inflammatory properties.

I'll admit that I went overboard when I first discovered chia seeds. I made chia pudding, which could have served as a science experiment. The texture was unique. Let's just say it took a few attempts to perfect the recipe. Now I add chia seeds to yogurt, smoothies, and even jam.

7. Olive Oil is Liquid Gold

Extra virgin olive oil is a Mediterranean diet staple, known for its anti-inflammatory and heart-protective properties. It's versatile, tasty, and, let's be honest, makes you feel like a chef even if you're just drizzling it over salad.

My first experience with high-quality olive oil was a revelation. I drizzled it on a slice of crusty bread, sprinkled with sea salt, and took a bite. I felt like I was dining in Italy (despite the fact that I was standing in my kitchen in sweatpants). Now, olive oil is my go-to for cooking, salad dressing, and even vegetable dip.

There were setbacks, such as accidentally using cayenne instead of paprika in a soup (hello, fire breath), as well as small victories, such as perfecting my turmeric latte recipe.

The point is that you don't need to be perfect. Experiment, laugh at your mistakes, and enjoy your successes. These powerhouses are more than just foods; they're tools for feeling your best. Who knew fighting inflammation could be so delicious (and entertaining)?

Allowed Foods

1. Vegetables (Rich in Vitamins, Minerals, and Fiber):
- Leafy Greens: Kale, spinach, Swiss chard, collard greens
- Cruciferous Vegetables: Broccoli, cauliflower, Brussels sprouts, cabbage
- Colorful Veggies: Bell peppers, carrots, sweet potatoes, zucchini, beets

- Alliums: Garlic, onions, leeks

2. Fruits (Antioxidant Powerhouses):
- Berries: Blueberries, strawberries, raspberries, blackberries
- Citrus: Oranges, lemons, limes, grapefruits
- Tropical Fruits: Pineapple, mango, papaya
- Apples, pears, cherries, and grapes

3. Healthy Fats:
- Olive oil (extra virgin preferred)
- Avocado and avocado oil
- Nuts: Almonds, walnuts, pistachios
- Seeds: Chia seeds, flaxseeds, sunflower seeds, pumpkin seeds
- Fatty Fish: Salmon, mackerel, sardines, herring, tuna

4. Whole Grains (Unrefined and Gluten-Free):
- Quinoa
- Brown rice
- Oats (gluten-free if needed)
- Buckwheat
- Amaranth

5. Legumes (Plant-Based Protein):
- Lentils
- Chickpeas
- Black beans, kidney beans, pinto beans

6. Spices and Herbs (Anti-Inflammatory Boosters):
- Turmeric (with black pepper for absorption)
- Ginger
- Cinnamon
- Garlic
- Basil, oregano, thyme, rosemary

7. Beverages:
- Green tea
- Herbal teas (chamomile, ginger, turmeric)
- Bone broth
- Water (plain or infused with fruits/veggies)

8. Proteins:
- Grass-fed, organic, or pastured meats (in moderation)
- Free-range poultry (chicken, turkey)
- Organic eggs
- Plant-based proteins like tofu and tempeh

9. Dairy Alternatives:

- Unsweetened almond milk, coconut milk, or oat milk

10. Sweeteners (Used Sparingly):
- Raw honey
- Pure maple syrup
- Coconut sugar

Not Allowed Foods (Inflammation Promoters)

1. Processed Foods:
- Packaged snacks (chips, crackers, cookies)
- Fast food
- Frozen dinners with additives and preservatives

2. Refined Sugars and Artificial Sweeteners:
- Table sugar, high-fructose corn syrup
- Artificial sweeteners like aspartame, sucralose

3. Refined Carbohydrates:
- White bread, white rice, white pasta
- Pastries, cakes, and muffins made with refined flour

4. Fried and Processed Oils:
- Vegetable oils: Canola, soybean, sunflower, corn oil
- Margarine and shortening

5. Red and Processed Meats:
- Sausages, bacon, hot dogs, deli meats
- Factory-farmed beef and pork

6. Dairy Products (For Some):
- Milk, cream, cheese (especially highly processed ones)
- Yogurts with added sugars

7. Beverages:
- Sugary drinks (sodas, sweetened teas, energy drinks)
- Alcohol (especially beer and sugary cocktails)

8. Artificial Additives and Preservatives:
- Monosodium glutamate (MSG)
- Artificial colors and flavors
- Nitrates and nitrites

9. Trans Fats:
- Hydrogenated oils
- Processed baked goods (store-bought cookies, cakes, etc.)

10. Excess Salt:
- Highly salted snacks
- Packaged soups and canned foods with high sodium

Notes for Individual Adjustments

- Food Sensitivities: Some individuals may need to avoid gluten, nightshades (like tomatoes, potatoes, peppers, and eggplants), or legumes if they exacerbate symptoms.

2: BREAKFAST AND BRUNCH

Scrambled eggs with sumac

Serves 2 Prep Time: 5 minutes Cooking Time: 5 minutes

4 large pasture-raised eggs
1 tablespoon avocado oil or olive oil
1 tablespoon pine nuts
1/2 teaspoon ground sumac
1 tablespoon fresh parsley, chopped
1/4 teaspoon sea salt
1/4 teaspoon black pepper
A squeeze of fresh lemon juice for added tang

1. To toast the pine nuts, heat a small, dry skillet over medium heat.
Toast the pine nuts for 1-2 minutes, stirring frequently, until they are golden brown and fragrant. Remove from the heat and set aside.

2. Prepare the scrambled eggs. In a medium mixing bowl, combine the eggs, sea salt, black pepper (if using), and ground sumac until well combined.
Heat the avocado oil in a nonstick skillet over medium heat.
Pour in the egg mixture and cook, stirring gently with a spatula, until soft and scrambled (about 2-3 minutes).

3. Remove skillet from heat and add toasted pine nuts and fresh parsley.
If desired, add a squeeze of lemon juice to boost the brightness.

4. Plate the scrambled eggs and garnish with extra parsley or pine nuts. Serve

Tofu shakshuka

Serves 4 Prep Time: 10 minutes Cooking Time: 20 minutes

1 tablespoon avocado oil or olive oil
1 onion, finely diced
1 red bell pepper, diced
2 cloves garlic, minced
1 teaspoon ground cumin
1 teaspoon smoked paprika
1/2 teaspoon ground turmeric
1/4 teaspoon ground cinnamon
1 can (14 oz) diced tomatoes, no added salt
1/4 cup tomato paste
1/2 cup water or vegetable broth (low-sodium)
1 block (14 oz) firm tofu, drained and crumbled
1/2 teaspoon sea salt or to taste
1/4 teaspoon black pepper
1 tablespoon fresh parsley, chopped
1 tablespoon fresh cilantro, chopped
a drizzle of tahini, a sprinkle of sesame seeds, or avocado slices

1. To prepare the sauce, heat avocado oil in a large skillet over medium heat.
Sauté the onion and red bell pepper for 5-6 minutes, until softened.
Cook for an additional 1-2 minutes, stirring in the garlic, cumin, smoked paprika, turmeric, and cinnamon until fragrant.

2. Create the Shakshuka base
Mix in the diced tomatoes and tomato paste. Bring the water or vegetable broth to a simmer.
Reduce the heat and cook for 10 minutes, stirring occasionally, until the sauce has thickened. Season with sea salt and black pepper to taste.

3. Gently crumble the tofu into the sauce and stir to combine. Continue cooking for an additional 5-7 minutes to allow the tofu to absorb the sauce's flavors.

4. Remove from heat and garnish with fresh parsley and cilantro.
Optional: Drizzle with tahini, sprinkle with sesame seeds, or top with avocado slices for added richness.

Tofu scramble on corn tortilla with salsa

Serves 2 Prep Time: 10 minutes Cooking Time: 10 minutes

1 tablespoon avocado oil or olive oil
1/2 small onion, diced
1 small bell pepper, diced
1/2 teaspoon ground turmeric
1/2 teaspoon smoked paprika
1/4 teaspoon black pepper
1/4 teaspoon sea salt

1 block (about 200g) firm tofu, drained and crumbled
2 small corn tortillas
1/2 cup fresh salsa
fresh cilantro, avocado slices, lime wedges

1. Prepare the Tofu Scramble. Heat the avocado oil in a medium skillet over medium heat.
Cook the diced onion and bell pepper for 3-4 minutes, or until softened.
Combine the turmeric, smoked paprika, black pepper, and sea salt. Cook for an additional minute, allowing the spices to toast and become fragrant.
Add the crumbled tofu to the skillet and combine with the vegetables and spices. Cook for 5-6 minutes, stirring occasionally, until the tofu is heated through and lightly golden.

2. Prepare the salsa. In a small bowl, mix together fresh diced tomatoes, cilantro, red onion, lime juice, and a pinch of sea salt. Adjust the seasoning to your taste.

3. Cook corn tortillas in a dry skillet over medium heat for 30 seconds per side, or until soft and slightly golden.

4. Assemble the dish by placing each warm tortilla on a plate and spooning the tofu scramble evenly into the center.
Top with the fresh salsa and any other desired toppings, such as avocado slices or cilantro.

5. Serve with lime wedges on the side to add freshness.

Buckwheat and chia seed porridge

Serves 2 Prep Time: 5 minutes Cooking Time: 15 minutes

1/2 cup buckwheat groats or buckwheat flakes
1 tablespoon chia seeds
1 1/2 cups unsweetened almond milk or coconut milk
1 tablespoon maple syrup
1/2 teaspoon ground cinnamon
1/4 teaspoon ground turmeric
1/4 teaspoon sea salt
1/2 teaspoon vanilla extract
1/4 cup fresh or frozen berries (blueberries, strawberries, raspberries)
nuts (walnuts, almonds), seeds (pumpkin or sunflower), and a drizzle of honey

1. Cook the buckwheat. In a medium saucepan, mix the buckwheat groats, chia seeds, almond milk, cinnamon, turmeric (if using), and sea salt.
Bring to a simmer on medium heat, stirring occasionally.
Reduce the heat to low and cook for 12-15 minutes, stirring occasionally, until the buckwheat is tender and the porridge has thickened.

2. Once porridge reaches desired consistency, remove from heat and add vanilla extract and maple syrup (optional).

3. To serve, spoon the porridge into bowls and top with fresh or frozen berries, nuts, or seeds.

Oat porridge with berries

Serves 2 Prep Time: 5 minutes Cooking Time: 10 minutes

1 cup rolled oats
2 cups unsweetened almond milk or coconut milk
1 tablespoon chia seeds
1/2 teaspoon cinnamon
1/4 teaspoon turmeric powder
1/4 teaspoon sea salt
1 teaspoon pure maple syrup
1/2 teaspoon vanilla extract
1/2 cup mixed fresh berries
chopped nuts (e.g., almonds or walnuts), hemp seeds, or a dollop of coconut yogurt

1. Cook the Oatmeal In a medium saucepan, combine rolled oats, almond milk, chia seeds, cinnamon, turmeric (optional), and sea salt. Bring to a boil over medium heat, then reduce to a low heat and simmer for 5-7 minutes, stirring occasionally, until the oats are tender and the mixture has thickened to your desired consistency.

2. Add maple syrup (optional) and vanilla extract to the cooked porridge for added flavor.

3. Divide porridge into two bowls. Add mixed berries and any other toppings, such as chopped nuts, hemp seeds, or coconut yogurt, for texture and nutrients.

Breakfast burritos with refried beans

Serves 2 Prep Time: 10 minutes Cooking Time: 15 minutes

2 gluten-free or whole grain tortillas
1 tablespoon avocado oil or olive oil
1/2 onion, diced
1/2 bell pepper, diced
1/2 zucchini, diced
1/2 cup corn kernels (fresh or frozen)
1 cup cooked refried beans (preferably homemade or low-sodium canned)
4 large pasture-raised eggs
1/4 teaspoon cumin
1/4 teaspoon smoked paprika
1/4 teaspoon turmeric
1/4 teaspoon sea salt
1/4 teaspoon black pepper
Fresh cilantro, chopped
avocado slices, salsa, dairy-free sour cream, or a squeeze of lime

1. To sauté the vegetables, heat avocado oil in a large skillet over medium-high heat. Sauté the onion, bell pepper, zucchini, and corn for 5-7 minutes, until softened and slightly caramelized.
Combine the cumin, smoked paprika, turmeric (if using), sea salt, and black pepper. Set aside.

2. Prepare the refried beans. In a separate pan, heat the refried beans on low heat, stirring occasionally, until warmed through. If the beans are too thick, add a splash of water to achieve the desired consistency.

3. Cook the Eggs - In a small bowl, whisk the eggs and season with sea salt.
In the same skillet as the vegetables, scramble the eggs over medium heat until cooked through and fluffy, about 2-3 minutes.

4. To assemble the burritos, warm the tortillas in a dry skillet for 1-2 minutes or wrap them in a damp towel and microwave for 20-30 seconds.
Spread a generous spoonful of refried beans across the center of each tortilla.
Arrange the sautéed vegetables on top of the beans, followed by the scrambled eggs.

5. Roll the tortillas tightly and fold in the sides to seal the burrito.
Garnish with fresh cilantro and optional toppings like avocado, salsa, dairy-free sour cream, or a squeeze of lime.

Sheet pan cauliflower tacos

Serves 4 (8 tacos) Prep Time: 10 minutes Cooking Time: 30 minutes

1 medium head of cauliflower, cut into florets
1 tablespoon avocado oil or olive oil
1 teaspoon cumin powder
1/2 teaspoon smoked paprika
1/4 teaspoon turmeric powder
1/4 teaspoon garlic powder
1/4 teaspoon ground black pepper
1/4 teaspoon sea salt

8 small gluten-free corn tortillas or grain-free tortillas
1/2 cup red cabbage, shredded
1/4 cup fresh cilantro, chopped
1 lime, cut into wedges
diced avocado, salsa, coconut yogurt, or pickled red onions

1. Preheat the oven to 400°F (200°C).

2. To prepare the cauliflower, toss it in a bowl with avocado oil, cumin, smoked paprika, turmeric, garlic powder, black pepper, and sea salt until evenly coated.
Spread the cauliflower in a single layer on a large sheet pan, ensuring that the pieces are not crowded.

3. Roast Cauliflower: Roast for 25-30 minutes, flipping halfway through, until golden and crispy on the edges.

4. Prepare the Tacos - Warm the tortillas in a dry skillet over medium heat for 1-2 minutes on each side until soft and pliable.
Once the cauliflower is done, take it out of the oven and set it aside.

5. Add 2-3 spoonfuls of roasted cauliflower to each tortilla.
Top with shredded cabbage, fresh cilantro, a squeeze of lime, and any additional desired toppings.

6. Serve tacos, garnished with extra lime wedges for extra zest.

Blueberry, Banana and Muffins

Makes 12 muffins Prep Time: 10 minutes Cooking Time: 20-25 minutes

1 1/2 cups gluten-free rolled oats or oat flour
1/2 cup almond flour
1 teaspoon baking powder
1/2 teaspoon baking soda
1/2 teaspoon ground cinnamon
1/4 teaspoon sea salt
2 ripe bananas, mashed
2 large eggs or flax eggs: 2 tablespoons ground flaxseed + 6 tablespoons water

1/4 cup unsweetened almond milk (or any non-dairy milk)
1/4 cup maple syrup
1 teaspoon vanilla extract
1/2 cup fresh or frozen blueberries
2 tablespoons chia seeds
2 tablespoons avocado oil or melted coconut oil

1. Preheat the oven and prepare the muffin tin.
Preheat the oven to 350°F/175°C.
Line a 12-cup muffin tin with paper liners or lightly grease with avocado oil.

2. Combine dry ingredients in a large bowl, including oats, almond flour, baking powder, baking soda, cinnamon, and sea salt.

3. Combine all wet ingredients. In a separate bowl, combine the mashed bananas, eggs (or flax eggs), almond milk, maple syrup (if using), vanilla extract, and avocado oil. Whisk until smooth.

4. Combine wet and dry ingredients. Stir gently until just combined. Don't overmix. Gently fold in the blueberries and chia seeds (if using).

5. Fill the Muffin Tin - Divide the batter evenly into 12 muffin cups, filling each about 3/4 of the way.

6. Bake the Muffins: Bake for 20-25 minutes, or until a toothpick inserted into the center comes out clean and the muffins are golden on top.
Allow the muffins to cool in their tins for 5 minutes before transferring to a wire rack to cool completely.

Whole grain toast with egg

Serves 1 Prep Time: 5 minutes Cooking Time: 5 minutes

1 slice of whole grain or sprouted grain bread
1 large pasture-raised egg
1 teaspoon avocado oil or olive oil
1/4 teaspoon turmeric powder
1/4 teaspoon black pepper
Pinch of sea salt
parsley, chives, or basil
smashed avocado, tomato slices, or a sprinkle of nutritional yeast

1. Toast whole grain bread until golden and crisp. Use a toaster or a skillet over medium heat.

2. Heat avocado oil in a small nonstick skillet over medium heat.
Crack the egg into the skillet, taking care not to break the yolk.
Season the egg with turmeric, black pepper, and a pinch of sea salt.
Cook the egg for 2-3 minutes, until the white is fully set but the yolk is still runny (or longer if you prefer a fully cooked yolk).

3. Assemble the Toast: Place the toasted bread on a plate.
Gently place the cooked egg on the toast.

4. Garnish with fresh herbs and optional toppings such as smashed avocado, tomato slices, or nutritional yeast for added flavor.

Chia pudding topped with goji berries

Serves 2 Prep Time: 5 minutes (plus 4 hours or overnight to set)

1/4 cup chia seeds
3/4 cup unsweetened almond milk or coconut milk
1 tablespoon maple syrup or raw honey
1/2 teaspoon vanilla extract
1 tablespoon ground flaxseeds
1 tablespoon hemp seeds

2 tablespoons goji berries (dried)
1/4 teaspoon cinnamon or turmeric powder
fresh berries, a sprinkle of coconut flakes, or a dollop of almond butter

1. In a small bowl or jar, combine the almond milk, chia seeds, maple syrup (or honey), and vanilla extract. Stir thoroughly to avoid clumping.
Add a pinch of cinnamon or turmeric powder for extra anti-inflammatory benefits.

2. Cover the bowl or jar and refrigerate for 4 hours or overnight. This allows the chia seeds to absorb the liquid and thicken into a pudding-like texture.

3. Toppings: Just before serving, sprinkle ground flaxseeds, hemp seeds, and goji berries over the chia pudding.

4. Stir gently to incorporate toppings, or leave on top for texture and crunch. For added flavor, top with extra fresh berries or a dollop of almond butter.

Sprouted grain English muffins

Makes 6 muffins Prep Time: 15 minutes (plus 1 hour for rising) Cooking Time: 15 minutes

1 1/2 cups sprouted whole wheat flour
1/2 cup almond flour
1 tablespoon ground flaxseeds
1 teaspoon baking powder
1/2 teaspoon sea salt
1 tablespoon olive oil or avocado oil
1/2 cup warm water (about 110°F / 45°C)
1 tablespoon raw honey or maple syrup
1 1/2 teaspoons active dry yeast
1 tablespoon apple cider vinegar
1 tablespoon chia seeds
1 tablespoon sesame seeds

1. In a small mixing bowl, combine warm water, honey or maple syrup, and active dry yeast. Gently stir and allow to sit for 5-10 minutes, or until frothy and bubbly.

2. Make the dough. In a large mixing bowl, combine sprouted whole wheat flour, almond flour, flaxseeds, baking powder, sea salt, and chia seeds (if desired).
Combine the yeast mixture, olive oil or avocado oil, and apple cider vinegar with the dry ingredients. Combine until it forms a soft dough.

3. On a lightly floured surface, knead the dough for 5-7 minutes, adding more flour as needed, until smooth and elastic.
Form the dough into a ball and return it to the bowl. Cover with a damp cloth and let it rise in a warm place for about an hour, or until doubled in size.

4. Shape the Muffins. Punch down the dough and divide into six equal portions. Shape each portion into a round ball, then flatten slightly to form a muffin shape.
Place the shaped muffins on a baking sheet covered with parchment paper or a silicone baking mat. Cover with a clean cloth and let them rise for an additional 15-20 minutes.

5. While the muffins rise, heat a cast-iron skillet or griddle over medium heat.
Place the muffins in the skillet and cook in batches if necessary. Cook for 4-5 minutes per side, until golden brown and firm to the touch.

6. Let the muffins cool on a wire rack for 10 minutes before slicing.
Serve warm, with your favorite toppings like avocado, nut butter, or cinnamon and honey.

Avocado on sprouted grain toast

Serves 1 Prep Time: 5 minutes Cooking Time: 2-3 minutes (for toasting)

2 slices sprouted grain bread (gluten-free if needed)
1 ripe avocado
1 tablespoon extra-virgin olive oil
1/2 teaspoon lemon juice or to taste
1/4 teaspoon sea salt
1/4 teaspoon black pepper
red pepper flakes, fresh herbs (parsley, cilantro, or basil), pumpkin seeds, or a drizzle of tahini

1. Toast sprouted grain bread slices until golden brown and crispy, about 2-3 minutes.

2. While the bread is toasting, cut the avocado in half, remove the pit, and scoop out the flesh into a bowl.
Mash the avocado with a fork until it's smooth but still slightly chunky.
Combine the olive oil, lemon juice, sea salt, and black pepper (if using). Adjust the seasoning as needed.

3. Spread the mashed avocado evenly on the toasted bread.

4. Optional toppings include red pepper flakes, fresh herbs, or a sprinkle of pumpkin seeds for crunch. Serve

Avocado toast with Sriracha

Serves 2 Prep Time: 5 minutes

2 slices of gluten-free sourdough bread or sprouted grain bread
1 large ripe avocado, mashed
1 teaspoon lime juice or lemon juice
1/4 teaspoon sea salt
1/4 teaspoon turmeric powder
1 tablespoon tahini
1/2 teaspoon harissa paste or a pinch of cayenne pepper
1 teaspoon water (to thin the tahini drizzle)
hemp seeds, sesame seeds, microgreens, or a sprinkle of paprika

1. Toast gluten-free sourdough slices until golden and crisp.

2. Prepare the avocado spread. In a small mixing bowl, combine the avocado, lime juice, sea salt, and turmeric powder (if using) until smooth.

3. Prepare the spicy tahini drizzle. In another bowl, combine the tahini, harissa paste, and water until smooth and drizzle-able. To adjust the spice level, add more or less harissa.

4. Spread mashed avocado evenly on toasted bread.
Drizzle the spicy tahini sauce over the avocado.

5. Garnish with hemp seeds, sesame seeds, or microgreens (optional).

Blueberry buckwheat pancakes

Serves 4 (8 small pancakes) Prep Time: 10 minutes Cooking Time: 15 minutes

1 cup buckwheat flour
1 teaspoon baking powder
1/2 teaspoon cinnamon
1/4 teaspoon sea salt
1 large pasture-raised egg or flax egg: 1 tablespoon ground flaxseed + 3 tablespoons water
3/4 cup unsweetened almond milk (or coconut milk)
1 tablespoon maple syrup
1 teaspoon vanilla extract
1/2 cup fresh or frozen blueberries
1 tablespoon avocado oil
fresh blueberries, sliced banana, a drizzle of maple syrup, or a dollop of coconut yogurt

1. Prepare the batter. In a medium bowl, combine the buckwheat flour, baking powder, cinnamon, and sea salt.
In a separate bowl, combine the egg (or flax egg), almond milk, maple syrup, and vanilla extract.
Gradually combine the wet and dry ingredients, stirring until smooth. Take care not to overmix. Gently fold in the blueberries.

2. Cook the pancakes. Brush a thin layer of avocado oil onto a nonstick skillet or griddle set over medium heat.
Pour 1/4 cup batter into the skillet for each pancake.
Cook for 2-3 minutes, until bubbles appear on the surface and the edges begin to set.
Flip and cook for an additional 1-2 minutes, or until golden brown.
Repeat with the remaining batter, adding more oil to the skillet if necessary.

3. To serve, stack pancakes on a plate and top with toppings like blueberries, maple syrup, or coconut yogurt.

Scrambled egg with dill and feta

Serves 2 Prep Time: 5 minutes Cooking Time: 10 minutes

2 slices of gluten-free sourdough bread or sprouted grain bread
4 large pasture-raised eggs
2 tablespoons unsweetened almond milk or coconut milk
1 tablespoon avocado oil or olive oil
1 tablespoon fresh dill, chopped
1 ripe avocado, sliced or mashed
1/4 teaspoon sea salt
1/4 teaspoon black pepper
A sprinkle of nutritional yeast for a cheesy flavor

1. Toast gluten-free sourdough slices until golden brown.

2. Prepare the scrambled eggs. In a medium bowl, combine the eggs, almond milk, and sea salt.
Heat the avocado oil in a nonstick skillet over medium heat.
Pour in the egg mixture and stir with a spatula until soft and fluffy (about 2-3 minutes).
Stir in half of the chopped dill just before taking the eggs off the heat.

3. Assemble the Dish: Place the toasted bread on a plate.
Spread the mashed avocado on each slice, or top with avocado slices.
Place the scrambled eggs on top of the avocado.

4. Sprinkle the remaining dill over the eggs.
For an extra boost of flavor, sprinkle with nutritional yeast.

Smoked salmon, avocado, and poached eggs

Serves 2 Prep Time: 10 minutes Cooking Time: 10 minutes

2 slices of gluten-free bread (e.g., sprouted grain or almond flour bread)
1 ripe avocado, mashed
4 large pasture-raised eggs
1 tablespoon apple cider vinegar
4 ounces wild-caught smoked salmon (low-sodium)

1/4 teaspoon turmeric powder
1/4 teaspoon black pepper
Fresh dill or chives, chopped, for garnish
Lemon wedges for serving

1. To prepare the toast, toast the gluten-free bread until golden brown.
Mash the avocado in a bowl and season with turmeric powder and black pepper (if tolerated).

2. To poach the eggs, bring a medium saucepan of water to a gentle simmer. Include the apple cider vinegar (if using).
Crack an egg into a small bowl or ramekin. Swirl the simmering water with a spoon before gently sliding in the eggs one at a time.
Poach for 3-4 minutes, until the whites are firm but the yolks are still soft. Remove with a slotted spoon and transfer to a plate.

3. Assemble the dish by spreading the mashed avocado evenly on toasted bread slices.
Spread the smoked salmon over the avocado.
Top each slice with a poached egg.

4. Sprinkle with fresh dill or chives.
Finish with a lemon wedge on the side for a refreshing citrus twist.

Sautéed tomatoes and mushrooms

Serves 2 Prep Time: 10 minutes Cooking Time: 15 minutes

1 tablespoon avocado oil (or olive oil)
1 cup cherry tomatoes, halved
1 cup cremini mushrooms, sliced
1 clove garlic, minced
1 teaspoon turmeric powder
1/2 teaspoon smoked paprika

1/4 teaspoon black pepper
1/4 teaspoon sea salt
4 large pasture-raised eggs
Fresh parsley or basil, chopped, for garnish

1. Wash and slice cherry tomatoes and mushrooms. Mince the garlic.

2. To sauté the vegetables, heat 1/2 tablespoon avocado oil in a large skillet over medium heat.
Sauté the garlic for 30 seconds, until fragrant.
Add the mushrooms and cook for 4-5 minutes, or until softened.
Combine the cherry tomatoes, turmeric powder, smoked paprika, and a pinch of sea salt. Cook for an additional 4-5 minutes, stirring occasionally, until the tomatoes have softened and released their juices. Remove the mixture from the pan and set it aside.

3. Fry the eggs. In the same skillet, heat the remaining 1/2 tablespoon oil over medium heat.
Crack the eggs into the pan and cook until desired doneness. Sprinkle it with some sea salt.

4. Place the sautéed vegetables on two plates.
Garnish each serving with two fried eggs.
Garnish with fresh parsley or basil

3: PLANT-BASED MEALS

Stir-fried tofu and vegetables

Serves 4 Prep Time: 15 minutes Cooking Time: 10 minutes

1 block firm tofu, drained and pressed
1 tablespoon avocado oil or olive oil
1 cup broccoli florets
1 red bell pepper, sliced
1 small carrot, julienned
1 zucchini, sliced into half-moons
2 cloves garlic, minced
1 tablespoon fresh ginger, minced
2 tablespoons coconut aminos or tamari for gluten-free
1 tablespoon rice vinegar or apple cider vinegar
1 tablespoon sesame oil
1/2 teaspoon turmeric powder
1/4 teaspoon black pepper
1 tablespoon sesame seeds
Fresh cilantro

To prepare the lentil loaf, follow these steps:
1. Cook the lentils in a medium saucepan with water. Bring to a boil, then reduce to a low heat and cook for 20-25 minutes, until the lentils are tender. Drain the excess water and set aside to cool slightly.
2. Heat avocado oil in a large skillet over medium heat. Sauté the onion and garlic for 3-4 minutes, until soft. Cook for another 3-4 minutes, stirring occasionally.
3. In a large mixing bowl, combine cooked lentils, sautéed vegetables, oats, ground flaxseed, tomato paste, fresh herbs, and spices. Mix well.
4. Place the mixture in a loaf pan lined with parchment paper or greased with avocado oil. Push it down evenly.
5. Preheat the oven to 350°F/175°C. Bake for 35-40 minutes, or until the loaf is firm and lightly golden on top. Allow to cool for ten minutes before slicing.

To make the mushroom gravy, heat avocado oil in a saucepan over medium heat. Sauté the mushrooms first. Add the mushrooms and cook for 5-7 minutes, or until they release moisture and brown.
2. Cook the mushrooms for an additional 3-4 minutes, or until the onions and garlic are softened.
3. Combine the fresh thyme, tamari or coconut aminos, and vegetable broth, then bring to a simmer.
4. In a small bowl, whisk together the arrowroot powder and water to form a slurry. Slowly pour it into the simmering gravy, stirring constantly. Cook for an additional 3-5 minutes, until the gravy thickens. Season with salt to taste.

To prepare the roasted vegetables, first preheat the oven to 400°F (200°C).
2. In a large bowl, combine the mixed vegetables, avocado oil, turmeric, paprika, garlic powder, black pepper, and sea salt.
3. Place the seasoned vegetables on a baking sheet in a single layer. Roast for 25-30 minutes, stirring halfway, until golden brown and tender.

Prepare the Dish:
1. Cut the lentil loaf into six equal pieces.
2. Serve each slice with plenty of mushroom gravy and roasted vegetables on the side. Garnish with fresh parsley for extra color and flavor.

Grilled vegetable and pesto pasta

Serves 4 Prep Time: 15 minutes Cooking Time: 25 minutes

8 oz gluten-free pasta such as brown rice or chickpea pasta
1 tablespoon olive oil (for grilling)
1 medium zucchini, sliced
1 red bell pepper, sliced
1 small eggplant, sliced
1/2 cup cherry tomatoes, halved
1/4 cup pine nuts (toasted)
2 tablespoons fresh basil, chopped

For the Pesto
1 cup fresh basil leaves
1/4 cup extra virgin olive oil
2 tablespoons nutritional yeast
1/4 cup walnuts or sunflower seeds
1 clove garlic, minced
1 tablespoon lemon juice
1/4 teaspoon sea salt
1/4 teaspoon black pepper

1. Bring a large pot of water to a boil and cook the gluten-free pasta according to package instructions. Drain and set aside.

2. Preheat your grill or a grill pan over medium-high heat.
Toss the zucchini, bell pepper, eggplant, and cherry tomatoes with olive oil. Grill the vegetables for 4-5 minutes per side, or until they are tender and slightly charred. Remove from heat and set aside.

3. In a food processor, combine the fresh basil, olive oil, nutritional yeast (if using), walnuts or sunflower seeds, garlic, lemon juice, sea salt, and black pepper. Blend until smooth. Adjust the consistency with a little extra olive oil or water if needed.

4. In a large mixing bowl, toss the cooked pasta with the grilled vegetables.
Add the pesto and mix until everything is well coated.

5. Transfer the pasta to serving plates and sprinkle with toasted pine nuts and fresh basil for garnish. Serve

Black bean and sweet potato tacos

Serves 4 (2 tacos per person) Prep Time: 15 minutes Cooking Time: 25 minutes

For the Tacos:
2 medium sweet potatoes, peeled and diced
1 tablespoon olive oil or avocado oil
1 teaspoon cumin
1/2 teaspoon paprika
1/4 teaspoon chili powder
1 can (15 oz) black beans, drained and rinsed
8 small corn tortillas or gluten-free tortillas
1/4 cup red onion, finely diced
1/4 cup fresh cilantro, chopped
1 lime, cut into wedges

For the Avocado Cream:
1 ripe avocado
1/4 cup unsweetened coconut yogurt or regular yogurt if tolerated
1 tablespoon lime juice
1 tablespoon fresh cilantro, chopped
1/4 teaspoon sea salt
1/4 teaspoon black pepper

1. Preheat your oven to 400°F (200°C).
Toss the diced sweet potatoes with olive oil, cumin, paprika, chili powder, and a pinch of sea salt. Spread them out in an even layer on a baking sheet.
Roast the sweet potatoes in the oven for 20-25 minutes, or until tender and lightly caramelized, stirring halfway through.

2. While the sweet potatoes roast, place the avocado, coconut yogurt, lime juice, cilantro, sea salt, and black pepper in a blender or food processor.
Blend until smooth and creamy, scraping down the sides as needed. Adjust seasoning to taste.

3. In a small saucepan over medium heat, warm the black beans until heated through, about 3-4 minutes. Season with a pinch of cumin, paprika, and sea salt to taste.

4. While the beans are heating, warm the tortillas in a dry skillet over medium heat for about 30 seconds per side, or until soft and pliable.

5. Once the sweet potatoes are roasted, assemble the tacos by placing a scoop of black beans onto each tortilla.
Top with roasted sweet potatoes, a spoonful of avocado cream, diced red onion, and fresh cilantro.
Serve with lime wedges for extra freshness.

Thai red curry with tofu over rice

Serves 4 Prep Time: 15 minutes Cooking Time: 25 minutes

1 tablespoon avocado oil or coconut oil
1 block (14 oz) firm tofu, drained and cubed
1 medium onion, sliced
2 cloves garlic, minced
1 tablespoon fresh ginger, grated
1 red bell pepper, sliced
1 small zucchini, sliced
1 cup baby carrots, sliced
1 cup broccoli florets
1 can (14 oz) coconut milk (full-fat, unsweetened)
2 tablespoons Thai red curry paste (ensure it's free of additives like sugar)
2 tablespoons coconut aminos or tamari for a soy-free option
1 tablespoon lime juice
1 teaspoon turmeric powder
1/2 teaspoon ground coriander
1/4 teaspoon sea salt
1/2 cup fresh cilantro, chopped
Cooked brown rice or cauliflower rice for a low-carb option

1. To prepare the tofu, heat avocado oil in a large skillet or wok over medium heat. Cook the cubed tofu for 5-7 minutes, turning occasionally, until golden brown on all sides. Remove from the pan and set aside.

2. Sauté the vegetables in the same skillet, adding more oil as needed.
Saute the onion for 3-4 minutes, until softened.
Add the garlic and ginger and cook for another minute, or until fragrant.
Cook the bell pepper, zucchini, carrots, and broccoli in the pan, stirring frequently, for 5-7 minutes, or until tender but crisp.

3. Combine the red curry paste, turmeric, coriander, and coconut aminos. Cook for 2 minutes, until the spices become fragrant.
Add the coconut milk and bring the mixture to a gentle simmer.
Allow the curry to simmer for 5-7 minutes, until the flavors meld and the sauce thickens slightly.

4. Return the cooked tofu to the pan and stir to coat with curry sauce.
Stir in the lime juice and salt until thoroughly combined. Simmer for another 2-3 minutes to heat through.

5. Serve the curry with cooked rice or cauliflower rice.
Optionally, garnish with freshly chopped cilantro and a wedge of lime.

Garlic and chili veggie stir fry Noodles

Serves 2 Prep Time: 10 minutes Cooking Time: 15 minutes

1 tablespoon avocado oil or olive oil
2 garlic cloves, minced
1 red chili, deseeded and finely chopped
1 medium carrot, julienned
1 bell pepper, thinly sliced
1/2 cup broccoli florets
1/2 cup snap peas, trimmed
2 cups baby spinach or kale
1 tablespoon fresh ginger, grated
2 tablespoons coconut aminos or tamari for a gluten-free option
1 tablespoon rice vinegar or apple cider vinegar
1 teaspoon sesame oil
1/2 teaspoon turmeric powder
1 tablespoon fresh cilantro, chopped
1/2 cup cooked brown rice noodles or zucchini noodles (spiralized)
Sesame seeds for garnish

1. Prepare the noodles. If using brown rice noodles, cook according to the package directions. Drain and set aside. Spiralize zucchini noodles and set aside.

2. To sauté the vegetables, heat avocado oil in a large skillet or wok on medium-high heat.
Sauté the minced garlic and chopped chili for 1 minute, until fragrant.
Place the carrots, bell pepper, broccoli, and snap peas in the skillet. Stir-fry the vegetables for 5-6 minutes, until they are tender but still crisp.

3. Stir in spinach or kale and grated ginger, cooking for 1-2 minutes until wilted.

4. Season the stir-fry. Toss the cooked noodles into the skillet with the vegetables. Mix in the coconut aminos, rice vinegar, sesame oil, and turmeric powder. Mix well to ensure the noodles are evenly coated and heated through.

5. Remove from heat and transfer stir-fry to plates.
Optional garnishes include fresh cilantro and sesame seeds.

Couscous with chickpea and stew

Serves 4 Prep Time: 10 minutes Cooking Time: 25 minutes

1 cup whole wheat couscous or quinoa f
1 tablespoon avocado oil (or olive oil)
1 onion, finely diced
2 cloves garlic, minced
1 medium courgette (zucchini), diced
1 can (15 oz) chickpeas, drained and rinsed
1 can (14.5 oz) diced tomatoes, no added salt
1 cup vegetable broth (low-sodium)
1 teaspoon ground cumin
1 teaspoon ground turmeric
1/2 teaspoon ground cinnamon
1/2 teaspoon smoked paprika
1/4 teaspoon sea salt or to taste
1/4 teaspoon black pepper
1 tablespoon fresh lemon juice
2 tablespoons fresh cilantro, chopped
1/4 cup pomegranate seeds

1. Prepare the couscous. Cook the couscous according to the package directions (or rinse and cook the quinoa with twice as much water). After cooking, fluff with a fork and set aside.

2. Cook the stew. Heat the avocado oil in a large pot over medium heat. Sauté the diced onion for 5 minutes, until softened. Add the garlic and cook for another 1-2 minutes, or until fragrant.
Combine the diced courgette, chickpeas, diced tomatoes, and vegetable broth.
Combine cumin, turmeric, cinnamon, smoked paprika (if using), sea salt, and black pepper. Heat the mixture to a simmer.
Reduce the heat to low and simmer for 15-20 minutes, stirring occasionally, until the courgette is tender and the stew thickens slightly.

3. Add fresh lemon juice for a refreshing flavor. Serve the stew with couscous or quinoa.

4. To add color and antioxidants, garnish with fresh cilantro and pomegranate seeds. Serve.

Halloumi peanut curry

Serves 4 Prep Time: 10 minutes Cooking Time: 25 minutes

1 block (250g) halloumi cheese, cut into cubes
2 tablespoons coconut oil or avocado oil
1 medium onion, chopped
2 cloves garlic, minced
1 tablespoon fresh ginger, minced
1 tablespoon turmeric powder
1 tablespoon ground cumin
1 tablespoon ground coriander
1/2 teaspoon chili flakes
1 can (400g) full-fat coconut milk
1/2 cup natural peanut butter (smooth or chunky, preferably unsweetened)
1 cup vegetable broth (low-sodium)
1 cup diced tomatoes (fresh or canned)
1 cup spinach or kale, chopped
1 tablespoon fresh cilantro, chopped
1 tablespoon lime juice
1 tablespoon tamari or coconut aminos
Sea salt, to taste
Cooked brown rice or quinoa

1. To prepare the halloumi, heat 1 tablespoon coconut oil in a large pan or skillet over medium heat. Cook the halloumi cubes for 4-5 minutes, until golden and crispy on all sides. Remove the halloumi from the pan and set it aside.

2. Sauté the aromatics in the same pan with the remaining coconut oil.
Sauté the chopped onion for 3-4 minutes, until softened.
Cook for an additional 2 minutes, stirring in the minced garlic and ginger until fragrant.

3. Sprinkle with turmeric, cumin, coriander, and chili flakes (if using). Stir to coat the aromatic spices.
Add the coconut milk, peanut butter, vegetable broth, and tomatoes to the pan. Stir until well combined, then bring to a simmer.
Allow the sauce to cook for 10-12 minutes, stirring occasionally, until slightly thickened.

4. Add the Greens and Halloumi - Add the chopped spinach (or kale) and cook for 2-3 minutes, until wilted.
Gently fold in the crispy halloumi cubes, letting them absorb some of the sauce.

5. Add lime juice and tamari (or coconut aminos) to finish the curry. Season with sea salt to taste.

6. Serve the curry with cooked brown rice or quinoa for a complete meal.
Garnish with fresh cilantro and a squeeze of lime if desired.

Chickpea Mayo

Makes 1 cup Prep Time: 5 minutes

1 cup cooked chickpeas or 1 can, drained and rinsed
2 tablespoons tahini or sunflower seed butter for nut-free
2 tablespoons apple cider vinegar
1 tablespoon Dijon mustard
1/4 teaspoon turmeric powder
1/4 teaspoon garlic powder
1/4 teaspoon sea salt
1/4 teaspoon black pepper
1/3 cup extra virgin olive oil
Water, as needed

1. Blend the chickpeas. In a food processor or blender, mix together the chickpeas, tahini, apple cider vinegar, Dijon mustard, turmeric powder, garlic powder, sea salt, and black pepper (if using).
Blend until smooth, scraping the sides as necessary.

2. Slowly drizzle in olive oil while the processor runs. Continue to blend until the mayo reaches the desired creamy consistency. If the mayonnaise is too thick, gradually add a teaspoon of water until smooth.

3. Taste the mayo and adjust seasonings as needed. Add more salt, vinegar, or mustard to taste.

4. Transfer mayo to an airtight container and refrigerate for up to a week.

Chickpea curry

Serves 4 Prep Time: 10 minutes Cooking Time: 25 minutes

1 tablespoon coconut oil or avocado oil
1 small onion, diced
2 cloves garlic, minced
1-inch piece fresh ginger, minced
1 large tomato, chopped or 1/2 cup canned crushed tomatoes
1 can (15 oz) chickpeas, drained and rinsed
1 can (14 oz) full-fat coconut milk
1 cup vegetable broth or water
1 tablespoon ground turmeric
1 tablespoon ground cumin
1 teaspoon ground coriander
1 teaspoon ground cinnamon
1/2 teaspoon ground black pepper
1/2 teaspoon ground paprika
1/4 teaspoon cayenne pepper
1-2 cups spinach or kale, chopped
Salt to taste preferably sea salt
Fresh cilantro, chopped
Serve with quinoa, brown rice, or cauliflower rice

1. To sauté the base, heat coconut oil in a large pot or deep skillet on medium heat.
Saute the onion for 3-4 minutes, until softened.
Cook for an additional 1-2 minutes, stirring in the garlic and ginger until fragrant.

2. Mix in turmeric, cumin, coriander, cinnamon, black pepper, paprika, and cayenne pepper (if using). Cook for one minute, stirring constantly to toast the spices.

3. Stir in the chopped tomato (or canned crushed tomatoes) until well combined. Allow to cook for 3-4 minutes, until the tomato softens.
Place the chickpeas, coconut milk, and vegetable broth in the pot. Stir well and heat to a simmer.
Reduce the heat and let the curry simmer for 15-20 minutes, allowing the flavors to combine.

4. Stir in the chopped spinach or kale after the curry has thickened slightly. Taste and adjust the salt as needed.

5. Pour curry into bowls and top with fresh cilantro.
Serve on its own or alongside quinoa, brown rice, or cauliflower rice

Plant based vegetable frittata

Serves 4 Prep Time: 10 minutes Cooking Time: 20 minutes

1 tablespoon avocado oil or olive oil
1 small onion, diced
1 red bell pepper, diced
1 zucchini, sliced
1 cup spinach, chopped
1 cup broccoli florets, steamed or blanched
1/2 cup chickpea flour or other gluten-free flour
1 cup unsweetened almond milk or oat milk
1 tablespoon nutritional yeast
1 teaspoon turmeric powder
1/2 teaspoon garlic powder
1/2 teaspoon ground cumin
1/4 teaspoon black pepper
1/4 teaspoon sea salt
1 tablespoon fresh parsley, chopped
1 tablespoon fresh basil or oregano, chopped

1. Preheat the oven to 375°F (190° C).
Cook the avocado oil in a large oven-safe skillet over medium heat.
Sauté the onion, bell pepper, and zucchini for 5-7 minutes, until softened.
Cook the spinach for an additional 2 minutes, or until wilted. Stir in the steamed or blanched broccoli, then set aside in the skillet.

2. Prepare the chickpea mixture. In a medium mixing bowl, combine the chickpea flour, almond milk, nutritional yeast (if using), turmeric, garlic powder, cumin, black pepper, and sea salt. Whisk until smooth and thoroughly combined.

3. Assemble the frittata. Pour the chickpea mixture over the sautéed vegetables in the skillet, ensuring that they are evenly coated.
Allow the mixture to cook on the stovetop for 2-3 minutes until the edges are set. Then place the skillet in the preheated oven.

4. Bake for 15-20 minutes, or until firm and lightly golden on top. A knife inserted into the center should come out cleanly.

5. Let the frittata cool slightly before slicing. Garnish with fresh parsley, basil, or oregano. Serve warm or room temperature.

4: GRAINS AND PASTA

Teff and vegetable pilaf

Serves 4 Prep Time: 10 minutes Cooking Time: 30 minutes

1 cup teff (rinsed)
2 tablespoons olive oil or avocado oil
1 small onion, finely diced
2 cloves garlic, minced
1 medium carrot, diced
1 zucchini, diced
1 bell pepper, diced
1/2 cup frozen peas or fresh peas
1 teaspoon ground turmeric
1 teaspoon cumin
1/2 teaspoon ground cinnamon
1/4 teaspoon ground black pepper
1/2 teaspoon sea salt or to taste
2 cups vegetable broth (low-sodium) or water
1 tablespoon fresh parsley, chopped
1/4 cup toasted pumpkin seeds or slivered almonds for crunch

1. Cook the teff. In a medium saucepan, heat 2 cups vegetable broth or water to a boil.
Place the rinsed teff in the saucepan, reduce the heat to low, and cover.
Simmer for 15-20 minutes, or until the teff is soft and the liquid is absorbed. Remove from the heat and allow to sit for 5 minutes, covered. Fluff with a fork.

2. Sauté the vegetables while the teff cooks. Heat olive oil in a large skillet over medium heat.
Sauté the diced onion and garlic for 3-4 minutes, until the onion is translucent.
Cook the carrot, zucchini, and bell pepper in the skillet for an additional 5-7 minutes, or until tender.
Cook for another 2 minutes, stirring in the peas, turmeric, cumin, cinnamon, black pepper (if using), and sea salt to bring out the flavors.

3. After sautéing the vegetables, add the fluffed teff to the skillet.
Stir well to combine and heat for an additional 2-3 minutes.
Garnish with fresh parsley and toasted seeds or almonds.

4. Serve the teff and vegetable pilaf as a main dish or side dish, paired with grilled chicken, fish, or tofu.

Red rice Mexican bowl

Serves 4 Prep Time: 15 minutes Cooking Time: 25 minutes

1 cup red rice or brown rice
2 tablespoons avocado oil or olive oil
1 small onion, diced
1 bell pepper, diced
2 cloves garlic, minced
1 teaspoon ground cumin
1/2 teaspoon smoked paprika
1/4 teaspoon ground turmeric
1/4 teaspoon sea salt
1/4 teaspoon black pepper
1 cup black beans (cooked or canned, drained and rinsed)
1 cup corn kernels (fresh, frozen, or canned, drained)
1 large ripe avocado, diced
1/2 cup cherry tomatoes, halved
1/4 cup fresh cilantro, chopped
Juice of 1 lime
fresh jalapeños, salsa, dairy-free yogurt, or pumpkin seeds

1. Rinse the red rice thoroughly with cold water before cooking it. In a medium saucepan, combine the rice and two cups of water. Bring to a boil and then reduce to a simmer. Cover and cook for 20-25 minutes, until the rice is tender and the water has been absorbed. Fluff with a fork, then set aside.

2. Sauté the vegetables while the rice cooks. Heat avocado oil in a large skillet over medium heat. Cook the diced onion and bell pepper for 5-7 minutes, or until softened.
Stir in the garlic, cumin, smoked paprika, turmeric, sea salt, and black pepper until fragrant, about 1 minute.

3. Stir in the black beans and corn, cooking for 3-4 minutes until fully heated.

4. Divide cooked rice into four bowls. Top with sautéed vegetables, diced avocado, halved cherry tomatoes, and a sprinkle of fresh cilantro.
Squeeze lime juice on top for extra flavor.

5. Serve Optional toppings include sliced jalapeños for heat, salsa, dairy-free yogurt, or pumpkin seeds for crunch. Serve immediately.

Amaranth porridge bowl

Serves 2 Prep Time: 5 minutes Cooking Time: 20 minutes

1/2 cup amaranth grains
1 cup unsweetened almond milk or coconut milk
1/2 cup water
1/2 teaspoon ground cinnamon
1/4 teaspoon turmeric powder
1 tablespoon maple syrup or raw honey
1 tablespoon chia seeds
1/4 teaspoon sea salt
1/4 cup fresh or dried blueberries
1 tablespoon pumpkin seeds or sliced almonds
1/2 ripe avocado, sliced
1 tablespoon shredded coconut (unsweetened)

1. Rinse with cold water and drain.
In a medium saucepan, mix together the rinsed amaranth, almond milk, water, cinnamon, turmeric, and sea salt.
Bring to a gentle simmer over medium heat, stirring occasionally. Once the mixture begins to boil, reduce the heat to low and cover the saucepan. Allow it to simmer for about 15-20 minutes, or until the amaranth softens and the liquid is absorbed.

2. Once the amaranth is cooked, add maple syrup or honey as desired.
If using, add the chia seeds and mix thoroughly. Allow the mixture to sit for a minute or two so that the chia seeds can hydrate.

3. Spoon porridge into bowls.
Garnish each bowl with fresh or dried blueberries, sliced avocado, pumpkin seeds or almonds, and shredded coconut.

Black rice Asian bowl

Serves 2 Prep Time: 15 minutes Cooking Time: 25 minutes

1/2 cup black rice (rinsed)
1 cup water or vegetable broth
1 tablespoon avocado oil or sesame oil
1 small carrot, julienned
1/2 cucumber, thinly sliced
1/4 cup red cabbage, shredded
1/4 cup edamame (fresh or thawed if frozen)
1 tablespoon fresh cilantro, chopped
1 tablespoon sesame seeds

For the Dressing
1 tablespoon tamari (gluten-free soy sauce)
1 tablespoon rice vinegar
1 teaspoon sesame oil
1 teaspoon grated fresh ginger
1 teaspoon honey or maple syrup
1/2 teaspoon turmeric powder
1/4 teaspoon black pepper

1. Cook the black rice. In a medium saucepan, heat 1 cup water or vegetable broth to a boil. Add the black rice, reduce the heat to low, and cover. Simmer for 25 minutes, until the rice is tender and the water has been absorbed. Remove from heat and let sit for 5 minutes before fluffing with a fork.

2. Begin preparing the vegetables while the rice cooks. Julienne the carrot, slice the cucumber, and shred the red cabbage. Set aside. – If using frozen edamame, rinse and thaw thoroughly in warm water.

3. In a small bowl, combine the tamari, rice vinegar, sesame oil, grated ginger, honey, turmeric, and black pepper. Whisk until smooth.

4. Assemble the Bowl: Divide cooked black rice between two bowls.
Place the carrot, cucumber, red cabbage, and edamame around the rice in each bowl.

5. Drizzle dressing over vegetables and rice. Garnish with chopped cilantro and sesame seeds. Serve

Millet Mediterranean bowl

Serves 2 Prep Time: 15 minutes Cooking Time: 20 minutes

1 cup millet, rinsed
2 cups water or vegetable broth
1 tablespoon extra-virgin olive oil
1/2 cup cucumber, diced
1/2 cup cherry tomatoes, halved
1/4 cup red onion, finely diced
1/4 cup kalamata olives, pitted and sliced
1/4 cup fresh parsley, chopped
1 tablespoon fresh mint, chopped

1 tablespoon tahini
1 tablespoon lemon juice
1/2 teaspoon ground cumin
1/4 teaspoon turmeric powder
1/4 teaspoon sea salt
Freshly ground black pepper

1. Cook the millet. In a medium saucepan, heat 2 cups of water or vegetable broth until boiling.
Add the rinsed millet, lower the heat to low, and cover.
Simmer for 15-20 minutes, until the liquid has been absorbed and the millet is tender.
Fluff with a fork, then remove from heat.

2. Prepare bowl ingredients: dice cucumber, halve cherry tomatoes, and finely chop red onion while millet cooks.
Slice the kalamata olives, and chop the parsley and mint.

3. In a small bowl, combine the tahini, lemon juice, cumin, turmeric, sea salt, and black pepper.
To thin the dressing to the desired consistency, add 1-2 tablespoons of water.

4. Assemble the Mediterranean Bowl by dividing the cooked millet into two bowls.
Place the cucumbers, tomatoes, red onion, olives, and fresh herbs on top of the millet.

5. Drizzle tahini dressing over bowls and serve

Wild rice and mushroom bowl

Serves 4 Prep Time: 10 minutes Cooking Time: 40 minutes

1 cup wild rice
2 cups low-sodium vegetable broth or water
2 tablespoons avocado oil or olive oil
1 medium onion, finely diced
2 garlic cloves, minced
8 ounces cremini mushrooms, sliced or a mix of wild mushrooms
1 teaspoon turmeric powder
1/2 teaspoon smoked paprika
1/4 teaspoon black pepper
1/4 teaspoon sea salt
2 cups fresh spinach, chopped
1/4 cup fresh parsley, chopped
2 tablespoons pumpkin seeds

1. Rinse thoroughly with cold water. In a medium saucepan, combine the wild rice with the vegetable broth. Bring to a boil, then reduce to a simmer. Cover and cook for 35-40 minutes, or until the rice is tender and the liquid has been absorbed.

2. To sauté the vegetables, heat avocado oil in a large skillet over medium heat.
Sauté the diced onion for 3-4 minutes, until translucent.
Stir in the garlic and cook for another minute, until fragrant.
Add the mushrooms, turmeric powder, smoked paprika, black pepper, and sea salt. Cook for 6–8 minutes, stirring occasionally, until the mushrooms are tender and golden.

3. Cook the chopped spinach in the skillet with the mushrooms for 2-3 minutes until wilted.

4. Assemble the Bowl: Divide cooked wild rice among four bowls.
Top each bowl with the mushroom and spinach mixture.
Garnish with fresh parsley and pumpkin seeds for extra crunch and nutrients.

5. Serve warm as a meal or with roasted sweet potatoes or a simple green salad.

Chickpea rice pasta primavera

Serves 4 Prep Time: 15 minutes Cooking Time: 20 minutes

8 ounces chickpea or brown rice pasta
1 tablespoon avocado oil or olive oil
2 garlic cloves, minced
1 small onion, finely chopped
1 cup broccoli florets
1 cup zucchini, thinly sliced
1 cup cherry tomatoes, halved
1/2 cup bell peppers (any color), julienned
1/2 cup carrots, thinly sliced
1 teaspoon dried oregano
1 teaspoon dried basil
1/4 teaspoon turmeric powder
1/4 teaspoon sea salt
1/4 teaspoon black pepper
1/4 cup unsweetened almond milk or coconut milk
1/4 cup nutritional yeast
Juice of 1/2 lemon
Fresh parsley or basil

1. Cook the pasta. Bring a large pot of salted water to a boil, then cook the chickpea or brown rice pasta according to package directions. Drain and set aside.

2. To sauté the vegetables, heat avocado oil in a large skillet over medium heat.
Sauté the onion and garlic for 2-3 minutes, until fragrant.
Combine the broccoli, zucchini, bell peppers, and carrots. Cook for 5–7 minutes, stirring occasionally, until the vegetables are tender but still crisp.

3. Add tomatoes and seasonings. Add the cherry tomatoes, dried oregano, dried basil, turmeric powder, sea salt, and black pepper (if desired). Cook for an additional 2 minutes until the tomatoes soften.

4. To make the sauce, reduce heat to low and add almond milk and nutritional yeast to the skillet. Stir until the vegetables are fully coated with the creamy sauce.
Squeeze in the lemon juice and mix thoroughly.

5. Toss cooked pasta in a skillet until evenly combined and heated through.

6. Arrange in bowls or plates, garnish with fresh parsley or basil, and serve warm.

Lentil and brown rice pilaf

Serves 4 Prep Time: 10 minutes Cooking Time: 40 minutes

1/2 cup dry brown rice, rinsed
1/2 cup dry green or brown lentils, rinsed
1 tablespoon avocado oil or olive oil
1 small onion, finely diced
2 garlic cloves, minced
1 carrot, finely diced
1 celery stalk, finely diced
1 teaspoon turmeric powder
1/2 teaspoon cumin powder
1/4 teaspoon cinnamon
2 cups low-sodium vegetable broth or water
1/4 teaspoon sea salt
1/4 teaspoon black pepper
2 tablespoons fresh parsley or cilantro, chopped
toasted almonds, pumpkin seeds, or a squeeze of lemon

1. Prepare the lentils and rice. Place the rinsed lentils and brown rice in a medium bowl and set aside.

2. To sauté the vegetables, heat avocado oil in a large saucepan or skillet over medium heat.
Sauté the diced onion, carrot, and celery for 5-7 minutes, until softened.
Cook for 1 minute, stirring in the garlic, turmeric, cumin, and cinnamon, until fragrant.

3. Combine the rinsed lentils and rice in a skillet, stirring to coat with spices.
Pour in the vegetable broth and bring to a boil.
Reduce the heat to low, cover, and cook for 35-40 minutes, until the rice and lentils are tender and the liquid has been absorbed. Stir occasionally to avoid sticking.

4. Remove from the heat, season with sea salt and black pepper (if desired), and fluff with a fork.
Sprinkle with fresh parsley or cilantro and optional toppings such as toasted almonds or pumpkin seeds.

5. Serve warm as a main or side dish, accompanied by roasted vegetables or a green salad.

Mushroom And Garlic Quinoa Salad

Serves 4 Prep Time: 10 minutes Cooking Time: 20 minutes

1 cup quinoa, rinsed
2 cups water or vegetable broth (unsalted)
1 tablespoon avocado oil or olive oil
2 cups mushrooms, sliced (shiitake, cremini, or button)
3 cloves garlic, minced
2 cups fresh spinach, chopped

1/4 cup fresh parsley, chopped
2 tablespoons fresh lemon juice
1 teaspoon turmeric powder
1/4 teaspoon black pepper
1/4 teaspoon sea salt

1. Cook the quinoa. Heat water or vegetable broth in a medium saucepan until boiling. Add the quinoa, reduce the heat to low, cover, and cook for 15 minutes, or until fluffy. Remove from heat and cover for 5 minutes.

2. To sauté mushrooms and garlic, heat avocado oil in a large skillet over medium heat. Sauté the sliced mushrooms for 5-7 minutes, until golden brown and tender.
Add the minced garlic and cook for another 1-2 minutes, or until fragrant.

3. Combine cooked quinoa, mushrooms, and garlic in the skillet.
Add the chopped spinach and cook for 2-3 minutes, or until wilted.
Add the parsley, lemon juice, turmeric powder, black pepper, and sea salt. Toss to combine.

4. Serve warm or at room temperature, garnished with extra parsley or hemp seeds for added nutrients.

Farro Risotto with Butternut Squash

Serves 4 Prep Time: 10 minutes Cooking Time: 35 minutes

1 tablespoon avocado oil or olive oil
1 small onion, finely diced
2 garlic cloves, minced
1 cup pearled farro, rinsed
4 cups low-sodium vegetable broth, warmed
2 cups butternut squash, peeled and diced into small cubes
2 cups kale, stems removed and chopped
1/2 teaspoon turmeric powder
1/4 teaspoon smoked paprika
1/4 teaspoon sea salt
1/4 teaspoon black pepper
2 tablespoons nutritional yeast
2 tablespoons fresh parsley, chopped

1. Heat avocado oil in a large skillet or saucepan over medium heat.
Sauté the onion for 3-4 minutes, until softened. Add the garlic and cook for another 1-2 minutes, or until fragrant.

2. Stir the farro in the skillet with oil and aromatics. Toast for 1–2 minutes.
Pour in the warmed vegetable broth one ladleful at a time, stirring frequently. Allow the farro to absorb the majority of the liquid before adding another ladle.

3. After about 10 minutes of cooking, add butternut squash, turmeric, smoked paprika, sea salt, and black pepper.
Continue to stir in the broth until the farro is tender and the butternut squash is fully cooked (about 20 minutes).

4. Add chopped kale in the last 5 minutes of cooking. Cook until the kale has wilted but remains vibrant green.

5. Add nutritional yeast (if using) for a creamy, cheesy flavor. Seasonings can be adjusted as needed.

6. Divide the risotto into bowls and garnish with fresh parsley. Serve warm.

Spaghetti Squash with Asparagus

Serves 4 Prep Time: 10 minutes Cooking Time: 40 minutes

1 large spaghetti squash (about 2-3 pounds)
1 tablespoon avocado oil or olive oil
1 bunch asparagus, trimmed and cut into 2-inch pieces
1 clove garlic, minced
1 tablespoon fresh thyme leaves or 1 teaspoon dried thyme
Zest of 1 lemon
2 tablespoons fresh lemon juice
1/4 cup unsweetened coconut yogurt or a ricotta substitute like blended cashews
1/4 teaspoon sea salt
1/4 teaspoon black pepper
2 tablespoons nutritional yeast

1. Roast the spaghetti squash. Preheat the oven to 400 °F (200 °C).
Cut the spaghetti squash in half lengthwise, then scoop out the seeds.
Drizzle the cut sides with 1/2 tablespoon avocado oil and a pinch of sea salt.
Place the squash, cut side down, on a baking sheet lined with parchment paper and roast for 30-40 minutes, or until the flesh is tender and easily shredded with a fork.

2. While the squash roasts, warm the remaining 1/2 tablespoon avocado oil in a large skillet over medium heat.
Sauté the asparagus for 4-5 minutes, until tender and crisp.
Cook for an additional 1-2 minutes, stirring in the minced garlic and thyme until fragrant. Remove from heat.

3. Once the spaghetti squash is cool enough to handle, use a fork to scrape the flesh into strands.
Transfer the squash strands to the skillet alongside the asparagus. Stir in the lemon zest, lemon juice, and coconut yogurt until combined.
Season with sea salt and black pepper to taste.

4. Divide the mixture into bowls or plates. If you want a cheesy, nutty flavor, sprinkle it with nutritional yeast.
Garnish with extra thyme leaves and serve warm.

Spaghetti Squash Garlic Noodles

Serves 4 Prep Time: 10 minutes Cooking Time: 40 minutes

1 medium spaghetti squash (about 2-3 pounds)
2 tablespoons avocado oil or olive oil
4 garlic cloves, minced
1/4 teaspoon turmeric powder
1/4 teaspoon crushed red pepper flakes
1/4 teaspoon sea salt
2 tablespoons fresh parsley or cilantro, chopped toasted sesame seeds, chopped green onions, or a squeeze of lemon

1. Prepare the spaghetti squash. Preheat the oven to 400 °F (200 °C).
Cut the spaghetti squash in half lengthwise, then scoop out the seeds.
Brush the cut sides with 1 tablespoon of avocado oil, then place the squash halves cut side down on a baking sheet lined with parchment paper.
Roast for 30-40 minutes, or until the flesh is tender enough to shred with a fork.
Once slightly cooled, use a fork to scrape the strands into a large bowl and reserve.

2. Heat the remaining 1 tablespoon avocado oil in a large skillet over medium heat. Sauté the minced garlic for 1-2 minutes, until fragrant (but not burned).
Combine the turmeric powder, red pepper flakes (if using), and sea salt.

3. Cook the spaghetti squash in a skillet with garlic sauce. Toss gently to coat the squash with the sauce and heat for 2-3 minutes.

4. Transfer to a serving platter or individual bowls. Garnish with fresh parsley or cilantro, and add any additional toppings like toasted sesame seeds or green onions.

Spinach and chickpea curry with rice

Serves 4 Prep Time: 10 minutes Cooking Time: 25 minutes

For the Curry
1 tablespoon avocado oil or olive oil
1 small onion, finely diced
2 garlic cloves, minced
1-inch piece of fresh ginger, grated
1 teaspoon ground turmeric
1 teaspoon ground cumin
1 teaspoon ground coriander
1/4 teaspoon cayenne pepper
1 can (14 oz) coconut milk (unsweetened)
1 can (14 oz) chickpeas, rinsed and drained
3 cups fresh spinach, chopped
1/4 teaspoon sea salt
Juice of 1/2 a lemon
For the Rice
1 cup basmati rice, rinsed
2 cups water
Pinch of sea salt
Optional Garnishes
Fresh cilantro, chopped
Sliced green chili (if tolerated)
Lemon wedges

1. In a medium saucepan, heat 2 cups of water to a boil.
Combine the rinsed basmati rice with a pinch of sea salt. Cover and set the heat to low.
Simmer for 15 minutes, until the water has been absorbed and the rice is tender.
Remove from the heat and allow to rest for 5 minutes, covered.

2. Prepare the curry base. While the rice cooks, warm the avocado oil in a large skillet or pot over medium heat.
Sauté the onion for 3-4 minutes, until softened.
Stir in the garlic and ginger, cooking for 1 minute until fragrant.

3. Add the turmeric, cumin, coriander, and cayenne pepper (if using) to the skillet. Stir for 30 seconds to toast the spices.
Pour in the coconut milk and stir until well combined.

4. Add chickpeas and simmer for 10 minutes to let the flavors combine.
Stir in the spinach and cook for 2-3 minutes, or until wilted.
Season with sea salt and squeeze in lemon juice to brighten.

5. Fluff cooked basmati rice with a fork and divided among serving plates.

Serve the spinach and chickpea curry over rice.
If desired, add more lemon wedges and fresh cilantro to garnish.

5: SALADS AND LIGHT MEALS

Asian Slaw

Serves 4 Prep Time: 15 minutes

2 cups shredded purple cabbage
2 cups shredded green cabbage
1 large carrot, julienned or grated
1/2 red bell pepper, thinly sliced
1/2 cucumber, julienned
1/4 cup fresh cilantro, chopped
2 tablespoons sesame seeds (toasted)
1 tablespoon grated ginger
1 clove garlic, minced

For the Dressing:
3 tablespoons rice vinegar or apple cider vinegar
1 tablespoon tahini or almond butter
1 tablespoon maple syrup or honey
1 tablespoon sesame oil
1 teaspoon coconut aminos or tamari
1/2 teaspoon turmeric powder
1/4 teaspoon sea salt
1/4 teaspoon black pepper

1. In a large mixing bowl, combine shredded purple and green cabbage, julienned carrot, red bell pepper, cucumber, and chopped cilantro.
Toss the vegetables gently to mix.

2. Prepare the dressing In a small mixing bowl, combine the rice vinegar, tahini or almond butter, maple syrup or honey, sesame oil, coconut aminos, turmeric, sea salt, and black pepper.
Whisk until the dressing is smooth and thoroughly combined.

3. To make the slaw, pour the dressing over the vegetables and toss well to coat. Garnish with toasted sesame seeds and, if desired, fresh cilantro.

4. Allow 10-15 minutes for the slaw to meld flavors before serving.

Roasted Beet

Serves 4 Prep Time: 10 minutes Cooking Time: 50 minutes

4 medium beets, peeled and cut into 1-inch cubes
2 tablespoons extra virgin olive oil
2 cloves garlic, minced
1 teaspoon fresh thyme or rosemary
1/4 teaspoon sea salt
1/4 teaspoon black pepper
1 tablespoon balsamic vinegar
Fresh parsley, chopped

1. Preheat the oven to 400°F (200°C). Peel and cube the beets, placing them on a large baking sheet lined with parchment paper.

2. Drizzle the beets with olive oil and sprinkle with garlic, thyme, sea salt, and black pepper (if using). Toss the beets to ensure they are evenly coated with the oil and seasonings.

3. Roast the beets in the preheated oven for 45-50 minutes, or until tender when pierced with a fork. Halfway through, toss the beets to ensure they cook evenly.

4. Once roasted, remove the beets from the oven and drizzle with balsamic vinegar for a touch of acidity, if desired. Garnish with fresh parsley before serving.

Greek Chickpea

Serves 4 Prep Time: 10 minutes

2 cups cooked chickpeas or 1 can, drained and rinsed
1 cucumber, diced
1 cup cherry tomatoes, halved
1/2 red onion, thinly sliced
1/4 cup Kalamata olives, pitted and sliced
1/4 cup fresh parsley, chopped
1 tablespoon extra-virgin olive oil
1 tablespoon lemon juice
1 teaspoon dried oregano
1/4 teaspoon sea salt
1/4 teaspoon black pepper
1/4 teaspoon turmeric powder
1/4 cup crumbled feta cheese (omit for dairy-free version)

1. To prepare the salad, combine chickpeas, cucumber, cherry tomatoes, red onion, olives, and parsley in a large mixing bowl.

2. In a small mixing bowl, combine the olive oil, lemon juice, dried oregano, sea salt, black pepper, and turmeric powder (if using).

3. Toss the salad with the dressing until well coated.

4. Top with crumbled feta. Serve immediately, or chill for 30 minutes to allow the flavors to meld.

Kale and Sweet Potato

Serves 4 Prep Time: 15 minutes Cooking Time: 35 minutes

2 medium sweet potatoes, peeled and diced
1 tablespoon olive oil or avocado oil
1/2 teaspoon ground turmeric
1/4 teaspoon ground cumin
1/4 teaspoon smoked paprika
1/2 teaspoon sea salt or to taste
1/4 teaspoon black pepper

1 tablespoon olive oil
1 small onion, thinly sliced
2 garlic cloves, minced
6 cups kale, stems removed and chopped
1 tablespoon apple cider vinegar
1 tablespoon sesame seeds

1. Roast the Sweet Potatoes. Preheat the oven to 400 °F (200 °C).
Place the diced sweet potatoes on a baking sheet and drizzle them with 1 tablespoon of olive oil.
Season with turmeric, cumin, smoked paprika, salt, and pepper. Toss the sweet potatoes until evenly coated.
Roast for 25-30 minutes, flipping halfway through, or until sweet potatoes are golden and tender.

2. Sauté the Kale: In a large skillet, heat 1 tablespoon olive oil over medium heat while roasting the sweet potatoes.
Sauté the sliced onion for 5-7 minutes, until softened and slightly caramelized.
Add the minced garlic and cook for another minute, until fragrant.
Cook the chopped kale in the skillet, stirring occasionally, for 5-7 minutes, until wilted and tender. If the kale begins to stick, add a splash of water or vegetable broth to avoid burning.

3. After cooking the sweet potatoes and kale, combine them in a large bowl or on a serving platter.
To add flavor, drizzle with apple cider vinegar (if using) and gently toss to combine.
Sprinkle with sesame seeds for texture and nutritional value.

Lentil Tabbouleh

Serves 4 Prep Time: 15 minutes Cooking Time: 20 minutes

1 cup cooked green or black lentils or
1/2 cup dry lentils, cooked
1 cup finely chopped parsley
1/2 cup finely chopped mint leaves
1 cup diced cucumber (peeled, if desired)
1 cup diced tomatoes (seeds removed)
1/4 cup finely chopped red onion
3 tablespoons extra-virgin olive oil
2 tablespoons freshly squeezed lemon juice
1 clove garlic, minced
1/4 teaspoon sea salt
1/4 teaspoon black pepper
2 tablespoons toasted pumpkin seeds or hemp seeds

1. Rinse dry lentils thoroughly and cook in boiling water until tender (about 15-20 minutes). Drain and cool.

2. Prepare the vegetables: finely chop parsley, mint, cucumber, tomatoes, and red onion. Put them in a large mixing bowl.

3. Mix the dressing. In a small mixing bowl, combine olive oil, lemon juice, minced garlic, sea salt, and black pepper (if using).

4. Combine cooked lentils with vegetables.
Pour the dressing over the mixture and gently toss until well combined.

5. Transfer to a serving dish and garnish with toasted seeds as desired. Serve or chill for 30 minutes to allow the flavors to combine.

Lettuce wraps with smoked trout

Serves 2 Prep Time: 10 minutes

1 cup smoked trout, flaked
8 large butter lettuce leaves or romaine leaves, washed and dried
1/2 avocado, sliced
1/4 cup shredded carrots
1/4 cup cucumber, julienned
1/4 cup red bell pepper, thinly sliced
1 tablespoon fresh dill, chopped
1 tablespoon fresh parsley, chopped

1 tablespoon fresh lemon juice
1/2 teaspoon Dijon mustard
1 tablespoon olive oil
1/4 teaspoon black pepper
1/4 teaspoon sea salt

1. In a small mixing bowl, combine olive oil, lemon juice, Dijon mustard (if using), sea salt, and black pepper. Set aside.

2. Assemble the lettuce wraps. Place the lettuce leaves flat on a plate or work surface. Evenly distribute the smoked trout, avocado slices, shredded carrots, cucumber, and red bell pepper across each leaf.

3. Sprinkle dill and parsley over the filling.
Distribute the prepared dressing evenly over the assembled wraps.

4. Fold lettuce leaves to form wraps.

Chickpea egg salad wrap

Serves 2 Prep Time:10 minutes Cooking Time:10 minutes

1 cup cooked chickpeas or canned, rinsed and drained
2 pasture-raised eggs, hard-boiled and chopped
2 tablespoons unsweetened coconut yogurt or avocado-based mayo
1 teaspoon Dijon mustard
1/4 teaspoon turmeric powder
1/4 teaspoon sea salt
1/4 teaspoon black pepper
1/4 cup celery, finely diced
1/4 cup red onion, finely diced
1 tablespoon fresh parsley, chopped
2 large anti-inflammatory wraps (e.g., cassava or almond flour-based wraps)
1/2 cup baby spinach or mixed greens

1. Prepare the salad. In a medium mixing bowl, mash the chickpeas with a fork or potato masher until slightly chunky.
Combine the chopped hard-boiled eggs, coconut yogurt, mustard (if using), turmeric powder, sea salt, and black pepper. Mix until thoroughly combined.
Add the celery, red onion, and parsley for extra crunch and flavor.

2. To assemble the wraps, lay them flat on a clean surface.
Put a layer of baby spinach or mixed greens in the center of each wrap.
Place half of the chickpea and egg salad mixture on each wrap.

3. Fold the sides of the wrap inward and roll tightly.
Slice in half and serve right away, or wrap in parchment paper for an on-the-go meal.

Quinoa vegetable wrap

Serves 2 Prep Time:15 minutes Cooking Time: 15 minutes

For the Filling:
1/2 cup cooked quinoa
1 cup mixed vegetables (e.g., julienned carrots, zucchini, red bell pepper)
1/2 cup shredded purple cabbage
1 tablespoon avocado oil
1 clove garlic, minced
1/2 teaspoon turmeric powder
1/4 teaspoon cumin powder
1/4 teaspoon sea salt
1/4 teaspoon black pepper

For the Wrap:
2 large gluten-free tortillas or collard green leaves
1/2 avocado, sliced or mashed
1/4 cup hummus (homemade or store-bought, made without preservatives)

Optional Toppings:
2 tablespoons fresh cilantro, chopped
1 tablespoon sesame seeds or hemp seeds

1. If not already prepared, cook quinoa according to package instructions. Set aside.

2. To sauté the vegetables, heat avocado oil in a skillet over medium heat.
Add the garlic and cook for 1 minute, or until fragrant.
Combine the mixed vegetables and purple cabbage. Sauté for 5–7 minutes, or until slightly tender but still crispy.
Mix in the turmeric, cumin, sea salt, and black pepper (if using). Mix well and cook for an additional minute.
Remove from the heat and mix in the cooked quinoa.

3. Spread hummus on each tortilla or collard green leaf.
Spread mashed or sliced avocado on top of the hummus.
Spoon the quinoa and vegetable mixture onto the wrapper.
Garnish with fresh cilantro and sesame or hemp seeds as desired.

4. Roll the tortillas tightly, tucking in the sides as you go. If using collard greens, blanch them in hot water for 10-15 seconds to soften them before wrapping.
Cut each wrap in half and serve

Asian inspired rice paper rolls

Makes 8 rolls Prep Time: 20 minutes

For the Rolls
8 rice paper wrappers
1 cup purple cabbage, finely shredded
1 cup carrots, julienned
1/2 cup cucumber, julienned
1 avocado, thinly sliced
1/4 cup fresh mint leaves
1/4 cup fresh cilantro leaves
1/4 cup fresh basil leaves (Thai basil preferred)
1/2 cup cooked rice noodles

For the Dipping Sauce
2 tablespoons almond butter or tahini
1 tablespoon coconut aminos or gluten-free tamari
1 teaspoon sesame oil
1 teaspoon grated fresh ginger
Juice of 1 lime
1-2 tablespoons water

1. Wash and prepare all vegetables by slicing and julienning into thin strips.
2. Place them neatly on a plate for easy assembly.

3. Fill a large, shallow dish with warm water.
4. Soak one rice paper wrapper in water for 10-15 seconds until it softens.
5. Place the softened wrapper flat on a clean cutting board or damp towel.

6. Put a small handful of purple cabbage, carrots, cucumber, avocado slices, and herbs (mint, cilantro, basil) in the center of the rice paper.
7. If using rice noodles, place a small amount on top of the vegetables.
8. Fold the bottom of the wrapper over the filling, tucking in the sides and rolling tightly to seal.
9. Repeat for the remaining wrappers and filling.

10. In a small bowl, combine the almond butter, coconut aminos, sesame oil, ginger, and lime juice.
11. Add water, one tablespoon at a time, until the sauce reaches the desired consistency.

12. Place the rice paper rolls on a platter and serve with dipping sauce.

Mexican black bean lettuce wraps

Serves 4 Prep Time: 10 minutes Cooking Time: 15 minutes

1 tablespoon avocado oil
1 small red onion, finely diced
1 clove garlic, minced
1 cup cooked black beans (rinsed and drained if using canned)
1 teaspoon ground cumin
1/2 teaspoon smoked paprika
1/4 teaspoon turmeric powder
1/4 teaspoon chili powder
1/4 teaspoon sea salt
2 tablespoons fresh cilantro, chopped
8 large lettuce leaves (e.g., romaine, butter lettuce, or iceberg)

Toppings
1 avocado, diced or mashed
1/2 cup cherry tomatoes, diced
1/4 cup red bell pepper, finely diced
2 tablespoons green onions, sliced
Lime wedges for serving

1. Heat avocado oil in a medium skillet over medium heat.
Sauté the diced onion for 3-4 minutes, until softened.
Stir in the garlic and cook for 1 minute, until fragrant.
Mix in the black beans, cumin, smoked paprika, turmeric, chili powder (if using), and sea salt. Cook for 5 minutes, stirring occasionally, until the beans are warmed through and slightly softened.
Remove from the heat and mix in the fresh cilantro.

2. Prepare the lettuce wraps. Wash and pat dry the lettuce leaves. Arrange them flat on a serving platter.

3. Spread the black bean mixture evenly on lettuce leaves.
Top each wrap with diced avocado, cherry tomatoes, red bell pepper, and green onions.

4. Add fresh lime juice to the wraps before serving. Serve as a light, refreshing meal or snack.

Berry almond butter wrap

Serves 1 Prep Time: 5 minutes

1 gluten-free wrap or coconut flour tortilla
2 tablespoons almond butter (unsweetened, no added oils)
1/2 cup fresh mixed berries
1 teaspoon chia seeds
1 teaspoon raw honey or maple syrup
1/4 teaspoon cinnamon

1. Place the gluten-free wrap on a clean surface or plate.

2. Spread almond butter evenly across the wrap, leaving about an inch around the edges.

3. Sprinkle the mixed berries over the almond butter.
Add chia seeds (if using) and cinnamon

4. Drizzle raw honey or maple syrup over berries to add natural sweetness.

5. Roll the wrap into a burrito shape, tucking in the ends as you go.

6. Cut in half for easy handling

Rainbow lettuce boars

Serves 4 (8 boats) Prep Time: 15 minutes

8 large lettuce leaves
1 cup red bell pepper, julienned
1 cup yellow bell pepper, julienned
1 cup shredded purple cabbage
1 medium carrot, grated
1/2 cup cucumber, thinly sliced
1/4 cup fresh parsley or cilantro, chopped
1/4 cup toasted pumpkin seeds or sunflower seeds

For the Dressing
2 tablespoons tahini
1 tablespoon fresh lemon juice
1 tablespoon apple cider vinegar
1 teaspoon maple syrup
1/4 teaspoon turmeric powder
1/4 teaspoon sea salt
2 tablespoons water

1. Wash and dry the lettuce leaves. Place them flat on a clean surface.
Prepare the vegetables by julienning, shredding, and slicing as necessary.

2. In a small mixing bowl, combine the tahini, lemon juice, apple cider vinegar, maple syrup (if using), turmeric powder, sea salt, and water. Adjust the water to a smooth, pourable consistency.

3. Arrange lettuce leaves on a serving plate.
Arrange red and yellow bell peppers, shredded purple cabbage, grated carrot, and cucumber slices evenly across each leaf.

4. Drizzle tahini dressing over each lettuce boat.
To add crunch, sprinkle with fresh parsley or cilantro and toasted seeds.

Mediterranean hummus collard wrap

Serves 2 Prep Time: 15 minutes

4 large collard green leaves (washed, stems trimmed flat)
1 cup hummus (homemade or store-bought, avoid added oils or preservatives)
1/2 cup cucumber, thinly sliced
1/2 cup cherry tomatoes, halved
1/4 cup red onion, thinly sliced
1/4 cup Kalamata olives, pitted and chopped
1/4 cup shredded carrots
1/4 cup fresh parsley, chopped
1/4 cup fresh mint leaves
1/2 avocado, sliced
1/2 teaspoon sumac
1 tablespoon lemon juice

1. Prepare the collard leaves. To make the collard green leaves pliable, gently blanch them in boiling water for 20 seconds before immediately transferring to ice water to stop the cooking. Pat dry with a clean towel.

2. Assemble the Wraps: Place one collard green leaf flat on a cutting board, stem end facing you.
Spread 2-3 tablespoons of hummus evenly in the center of each leaf.
Place the cucumber, cherry tomatoes, red onion, Kalamata olives (if using), shredded carrots, parsley, mint, and avocado slices on top. Sprinkle with sumac (if using), then drizzle with lemon juice.

3. Fold the sides of the collard leaf inward and roll tightly from the stem end to form a burrito-style wrap. Repeat for the remaining leaves and ingredients.

4. Cut each wrap in half and serve immediately, or wrap in parchment for a portable meal.

Quinoa and citrus salad

Serves 4 Prep Time: 15 minutes Cooking Time: 15 minutes

1 cup quinoa, rinsed
2 cups water or low-sodium vegetable broth
1 cup mixed greens (e.g., arugula, spinach, or kale)
1 orange, peeled and segmented
1 grapefruit, peeled and segmented
1/4 cup pomegranate seeds
1/4 cup toasted walnuts or almonds
1/4 cup fresh mint leaves, chopped)

Dressing
3 tablespoons olive oil
2 tablespoons freshly squeezed lemon juice
1 tablespoon orange juice
1 teaspoon Dijon mustard
1/4 teaspoon turmeric powder
1/4 teaspoon sea salt
1/8 teaspoon black pepper

1. Cook the quinoa. In a medium saucepan, mix the rinsed quinoa with water or vegetable broth. Bring to a boil, then reduce heat to low, cover, and cook for 15 minutes, or until quinoa is tender and liquid has been absorbed. Fluff with a fork and allow to cool.

2. In a small mixing bowl or jar, combine olive oil, lemon juice, orange juice, Dijon mustard, turmeric, sea salt, and black pepper (if using). Set aside.

3. Assemble the salad. In a large mixing bowl, combine cooked quinoa, mixed greens, orange and grapefruit segments, pomegranate seeds, toasted nuts (if using), and fresh mint.

4. Pour dressing over salad and gently toss to coat.

5. Arrange salad on plates or bowls and serve

6: FISH AND SEAFOODS

Grilled mackerel with ginger

Serves 2 Prep Time: 10 minutes Cooking Time: 10 minutes

2 fresh mackerel fillets (about 6 oz each)
1 tablespoon fresh ginger, finely grated
2 garlic cloves, minced
2 tablespoons coconut aminos
1 tablespoon fresh lime juice
1 tablespoon avocado oil or olive oil

1/2 teaspoon turmeric powder
1/4 teaspoon ground black pepper
1/4 teaspoon sea salt
Fresh cilantro leaves
Lime wedges, for serving

1. Prepare the marinade. In a small mixing bowl, combine the grated ginger, minced garlic, coconut aminos, lime juice, avocado oil, turmeric powder, black pepper (optional), and sea salt.

2. Arrange the mackerel fillets in a shallow dish.
Pour the marinade over the fillets until they are evenly coated.
Cover and refrigerate for at least 15 minutes or up to an hour for a more intense flavor.

3. Preheat a grill or grill pan to medium-high heat.
To prevent sticking, lightly oil the grill grates or pan.
Place the marinated mackerel skin side down on the grill and cook for 4-5 minutes.
Cook for an additional 3-4 minutes, or until the fish flakes easily flaked with a fork.

4. Place the grilled mackerel on a plate and garnish with fresh cilantro leaves.
Serve with lime wedges on the side for an added burst of flavour.

Baked cod with Mediterranean flavors

Serves 4 Prep Time: 10 minutes Cooking Time: 20-25 minutes

4 fresh cod fillets (about 6 oz each)
2 tablespoons extra virgin olive oil
1 teaspoon dried oregano
1 teaspoon dried thyme
1 teaspoon garlic powder
1/2 teaspoon smoked paprika
1/4 teaspoon sea salt
1/4 teaspoon black pepper
1 tablespoon fresh lemon juice
1/4 cup Kalamata olives, pitted and chopped
1/4 cup cherry tomatoes, halved
1/4 cup red onion, thinly sliced
1 tablespoon fresh parsley, chopped
1 tablespoon capers

1. Preheat the oven to 375°F (190°C).

2. Dry the cod fillets with paper towels to remove excess moisture.
Put the fillets on a lined baking sheet or in a shallow baking dish.

3. Drizzle olive oil over fillets and gently rub to coat evenly.
Sprinkle the cod with dried oregano, thyme, garlic powder, smoked paprika, sea salt, and black pepper (optional).
To add brightness, squeeze fresh lemon juice over the fillets.

4. Scatter chopped olives, cherry tomatoes, red onion, and capers (if using) around the fish, leaving some vegetables on top.

5. Cook the cod in a preheated oven for 20-25 minutes, or until it flakes easily with a fork. Internal temperature should be 145°F (63°C).

6. Remove from the oven and top with fresh parsley. Serve immediately alongside your favorite anti-inflammatory side dishes, such as steamed broccoli, quinoa, or a leafy green salad.

Poached salmon with herbs

Serves 2 Prep Time: 5 minutes Cooking Time: 15 minutes

2 salmon fillets (6 oz each, wild-caught preferred)
2 cups water
1/2 cup white wine
1 tablespoon avocado oil or olive oil
1 small lemon, sliced
2 cloves garlic, smashed

1 teaspoon fresh dill, chopped
1 teaspoon fresh parsley, chopped
1/2 teaspoon sea salt
1/4 teaspoon black pepper

1. In a medium mixing bowl, combine the sliced heart of palm, avocado oil, smoked paprika, cumin, turmeric, garlic powder, sea salt, black pepper (optional), and lime juice.
Heat a nonstick skillet over medium heat, then add the seasoned heart of palm strips. Cook for 5–7 minutes, stirring occasionally, until slightly crispy and heated through. Remove from the heat and set aside.

2. In a large mixing bowl, combine the shredded cabbage, chopped cilantro, apple cider vinegar, olive oil, sea salt, black pepper (optional), and honey. Toss the cabbage until well coated, then set aside to marinate for 5 minutes.

3. In a small bowl, combine the coconut yogurt, minced chipotle in adobo or chipotle powder, lime juice, sea salt, and garlic powder. Stir until smooth. Adjust the seasoning to your taste.

4. To assemble the tacos, warm gluten-free corn tortillas in a dry skillet over medium heat for 1 minute on each side, until soft and pliable.
Spread a small amount of chipotle mayonnaise over each tortilla.
Add a generous serving of heart of palm "fish" strips, followed by a heap of cabbage slaw.
Garnish with fresh cilantro leaves and extra lime wedges if desired.

5. Serve tacos with extra chipotle mayo on the side for dipping.

Chickpea Tuna Salad Sandwich

Serves 2 Prep Time: 10 minutes

1 can (15 oz) chickpeas, drained and rinsed
1 can (5 oz) wild-caught tuna in water, drained
2 tablespoons olive oil or avocado oil
1 tablespoon lemon juice
1 teaspoon Dijon mustard
1/4 teaspoon turmeric powder
1/4 teaspoon sea salt
1/4 teaspoon black pepper
1/4 cup celery, finely diced
1 tablespoon fresh parsley, chopped
1-2 sheets nori, torn into small pieces
2 slices gluten-free bread or sprouted grain bread
leafy greens (e.g., spinach, arugula)

1. Prepare the Chickpea Tuna Salad.
In a large mixing bowl, mash the chickpeas roughly with a fork or potato masher, leaving some larger pieces for texture.
Add the drained tuna and gently combine.
Combine the olive oil, lemon juice, Dijon mustard (if using), turmeric powder, sea salt, and black pepper.
Gently mix in the diced celery, fresh parsley, and torn nori.

2. Toast gluten-free bread if desired, or use fresh bread for a softer texture.
Spread the chickpea tuna salad evenly across one slice of bread.
Top with the second slice of bread and any leafy greens you're using.

3. Cut the sandwich in half and serve

King Oyster Mushroom Scallops

Serves 2 Prep Time: 10 minutes Cooking Time: 15 minutes

2 large king oyster mushrooms
2 tablespoons avocado oil or olive oil
2 tablespoons grass-fed ghee or dairy-free butter
3 cloves garlic, minced
1 tablespoon fresh lemon juice
1 teaspoon fresh thyme or rosemary, chopped
1/4 teaspoon sea salt (to taste)
1/4 teaspoon black pepper
Fresh parsley, chopped

1. Trim the tough ends of the king oyster mushrooms and slice into thick "scallop-like" rounds, about 1 inch thick.
To remove moisture from the slices, gently pat them dry with a paper towel.

2. To cook the mushrooms, heat avocado oil in a large skillet over medium-high heat. When the oil is hot, add the mushroom slices and cook for 3-4 minutes per side, until golden brown and tender.
Remove the mushrooms from the skillet and set them aside.

3. In the same skillet, melt the ghee or dairy-free butter over medium heat.
Add the minced garlic and cook for 1-2 minutes, taking care not to burn.
Combine the lemon juice, fresh thyme or rosemary, sea salt, and black pepper.

4. Toss cooked mushrooms with garlic butter sauce for 1-2 minutes to absorb flavors.
Remove from heat and place the mushrooms on a plate.
Garnish with freshly chopped parsley and serve

Tofu Crab Cakes

Makes 6 cakes Prep Time: 15 minutes Cooking Time: 15 minutes

14 oz firm tofu, drained and pressed
1/2 cup almond flour or chickpea flour
1/4 cup finely chopped red bell pepper
1/4 cup finely chopped green onion
2 tablespoons fresh parsley, chopped
1 tablespoon Dijon mustard or yellow mustard
1 tablespoon lemon juice
1 teaspoon Old Bay seasoning
1/4 teaspoon turmeric powder
1/4 teaspoon smoked paprika
1/4 teaspoon sea salt
1/4 teaspoon black pepper
1 tablespoon avocado oil

1. Prepare the tofu. In a large mixing bowl, crumble the pressed tofu into small pieces with your hands or a fork.
Combine almond flour, red bell pepper, green onion, parsley, Dijon mustard, lemon juice, Old Bay seasoning, turmeric, smoked paprika (optional), sea salt, and black pepper. Mix until the ingredients are thoroughly combined. The mixture should hold together but be slightly crumbly. If the mixture seems too dry, add a teaspoon of water at a time until it comes together.

2. Divide the mixture into 6 equal portions and shape into 2-3 inch diameter patties.

3. Heat the avocado oil in a large skillet over medium heat.
Once hot, carefully place the patties in the skillet, making sure they are not too crowded. Fry for 3-4 minutes per side, until golden brown and crispy.
Remove the patties from the skillet and place on a paper towel to absorb any remaining oil.

4. Serve warm tofu "crab" cakes with mixed greens, dairy-free tartar sauce, or avocado salad.

Tempeh Fish Fillets

Serves 2 Prep Time: 15 minutes Cooking Time: 20 minutes

For the Tempeh "Fish" Fillets:
1 block of tempeh (about 8 oz), sliced into 1/2-inch thick fillets
1 tablespoon avocado oil or olive oil
1 tablespoon tamari or coconut aminos
1 teaspoon lemon juice
1/2 teaspoon dried thyme
1/4 teaspoon sea salt
1/4 teaspoon black pepper

For the Lemon-Dill Sauce:
1/4 cup coconut yogurt or unsweetened dairy-free yogurt
1 tablespoon fresh dill, chopped
1 tablespoon lemon juice
1 teaspoon Dijon mustard
1/2 teaspoon garlic powder
Pinch of sea salt

1. In a shallow dish, mix together tamari or coconut aminos, lemon juice, dried thyme, sea salt, and black pepper. Place the tempeh fillets in the marinade and soak for 5-10 minutes, flipping halfway to ensure both sides are coated.

2. Heat avocado oil in a skillet over medium heat.
Once hot, add the marinated tempeh fillets and cook for 3-4 minutes on each side, or until golden brown and slightly crispy.
Remove from the skillet and set aside while you make the sauce.

3. In a small mixing bowl, combine coconut yogurt, fresh dill, lemon juice, Dijon mustard (if using), garlic powder, and sea salt.
Stir the sauce thoroughly until it is smooth and creamy. Season to taste.

4. Plate tempeh fillets and drizzle with lemon-dill sauce. Optional garnishes include extra fresh dill or lemon wedges. Serve with steamed vegetables or a side salad to complete the meal.

Herb crusted halibut and mashed cauliflower

Serves 2 Prep Time: 10 minutes Cooking Time: 20 minutes

For the Herb-Crusted Halibut:
2 halibut fillets (about 6 oz each)
1 tablespoon avocado oil or olive oil
1 teaspoon dried thyme
1 teaspoon dried rosemary
1 teaspoon garlic powder
1/4 teaspoon sea salt
1/4 teaspoon black pepper
Juice of 1/2 lemon

For the Mashed Cauliflower:
1 medium head of cauliflower, cut into florets
2 tablespoons olive oil or avocado oil
1/4 cup unsweetened almond milk or coconut milk
1/2 teaspoon garlic powder
1/4 teaspoon sea salt
1/4 teaspoon black pepper
1 tablespoon fresh parsley, chopped

1. Prepare the mashed cauliflower. In a large pot, steam the cauliflower florets until tender, about 8-10 minutes. You can also microwave them in a covered bowl with a little water for 5-6 minutes.
Drain the cauliflower, then return it to the pot.
Season the cauliflower with olive oil, almond milk, garlic powder, sea salt, and black pepper. Using an immersion blender or a potato masher, blend until smooth and creamy. If necessary, increase the amount of almond milk to achieve the desired consistency.

2. Prepare the herb-crusted halibut. Preheat the oven to 375° Fahrenheit (190° Celsius).
In a small bowl, mix together the thyme, rosemary, garlic powder, sea salt, and black pepper.
Rub the halibut fillets with avocado oil, then coat with the herb mixture on both sides.
Heat a skillet over medium-high heat, then sear the fillets for 2 minutes on each side until golden.
Place the skillet in the preheated oven for 8-10 minutes, or until the fish flakes easily with a fork.

3. To serve, top the mashed cauliflower with herb-crusted halibut fillets.
Garnish with fresh parsley and a squeeze of lemon juice for added freshness.

7: SLOW COOKER OPTIONS

Golden Lentil & Sweet Potato Stew

Serves 6 Prep Time: 15 minutes Cooking Time: 4-6 hours (low) or 2-3 hours (high)

1 cup yellow lentils, rinsed
2 medium sweet potatoes, peeled and diced
1 medium onion, finely chopped
3 cloves garlic, minced
1 tablespoon fresh ginger, grated
1 teaspoon ground turmeric
1 teaspoon ground cumin
1/2 teaspoon cinnamon
1/4 teaspoon black pepper
4 cups low-sodium vegetable broth
1 (14-ounce) can full-fat coconut milk
2 cups fresh spinach, chopped
1 tablespoon avocado oil
1/2 teaspoon sea salt
Juice of 1/2 lemon
Fresh cilantro

1. Optional step for enhanced flavor: Sauté onion, garlic, and ginger in avocado oil over medium heat for 2-3 minutes.

2. Combine rinsed lentils, sweet potatoes, onion (sautéed or raw), garlic, ginger, turmeric, cumin, cinnamon, and black pepper in the slow cooker.
Pour in the vegetable broth and stir until combined.

3. Cover and cook on low for 4-6 hours or high for 2-3 hours, until lentils and sweet potatoes are tender.

4. Add coconut milk and spinach 15 minutes before serving. Allow the spinach to wilt while the stew heats through.

5. To serve, ladle the stew into bowls and garnish with lemon juice and fresh cilantro, if desired.

Moroccan Chickpea & Quinoa Soup

Serves 6 Prep Time:15 minutes Cooking Time: 6 hours (low) or 3 hours (high)

1 tablespoon olive oil
1 medium onion, diced
3 garlic cloves, minced
2 medium carrots, sliced into thin rounds
1 red bell pepper, diced
1 cup canned diced tomatoes (no salt added)
1 can (15 oz) chickpeas, drained and rinsed
1/2 cup uncooked quinoa, rinsed
4 cups low-sodium vegetable broth
1/2 teaspoon turmeric powder
1/4 teaspoon smoked paprika
1/2 teaspoon sea salt
1/4 teaspoon black pepper
1/4 teaspoon cayenne pepper
1 cup chopped fresh spinach or kale
Juice of 1 lemon
2 tablespoons fresh parsley or cilantro, chopped
1 teaspoon ground cumin
1 teaspoon ground coriander
1/2 teaspoon ground cinnamon

1. Optional: Sauté the aromatics with olive oil in a skillet over medium heat. Saute the onion, garlic, carrots, and red bell pepper for 3-4 minutes, until softened. (This step improves the flavor but can be skipped for convenience.)

2. Add ingredients to the slow cooker. Transfer the sautéed veggies to the slow cooker.
Mix in the diced tomatoes, chickpeas, quinoa, vegetable broth, cumin, coriander, cinnamon, turmeric, smoked paprika, sea salt, and black pepper (if using).

3. Cover and cook on low for 6 hours or high for 3 hours until the vegetables are tender and the quinoa is completely cooked.

4. Add greens and lemon juice. About 10 minutes before serving, add the spinach or kale and lemon juice. Let the greens wilt.

5. Ladle soup into bowls and top with fresh parsley or cilantro. Serve warm.

Mushroom & Brown Rice Congee

Serves 4 Prep Time: 10 minutes Cooking Time: 6-8 hours (slow cooker)

1 cup brown rice, rinsed
8 cups low-sodium vegetable broth or water
1 cup shiitake mushrooms, thinly sliced (fresh or dried)
1 tablespoon freshly grated ginger
2 cloves garlic, minced
1 tablespoon coconut aminos
1/4 teaspoon sea salt
2 cups bok choy, chopped
1 tablespoon sesame oil
2 green onions, thinly sliced
1 tablespoon sesame seeds

1. Rinse brown rice thoroughly with running water to remove excess starch. If using dried shiitake mushrooms, soak them for 15 minutes in warm water before slicing thinly.

2. Assemble in the slow cooker. Place the rinsed brown rice, vegetable broth, shiitake mushrooms, grated ginger, minced garlic, and coconut aminos in the slow cooker. Stir to combine.

3. Cover and cook on low for 6-8 hours or high for 3-4 hours, stirring occasionally if possible. The rice should break down into a creamy porridge-like texture.

4. Stir in chopped bok choy and sea salt in the final 15-20 minutes of cooking. Let it wilt and soften.

5. To serve, ladle the congee into bowls and drizzle with sesame oil if desired. Garnish with green onions and sesame seeds for extra flavor and crunch.

Butternut Squash & Apple Bisque

Serves 6 Prep Time: 15 minutes Cooking Time: 4-6 hours on low or 2-3 hours on high

1 medium butternut squash (about 3 lbs), peeled, seeded, and cubed
2 medium apples (such as Granny Smith or Fuji), peeled, cored, and chopped
1 small onion, diced
2 garlic cloves, minced
1 tablespoon fresh ginger, grated or 1 teaspoon ground ginger
1 teaspoon ground cinnamon
1/4 teaspoon ground nutmeg
1/2 teaspoon turmeric powder
4 cups low-sodium vegetable broth or filtered water
1 cup full-fat coconut milk
1 tablespoon fresh lemon juice
1/2 teaspoon sea salt
pumpkin seeds, a drizzle of coconut cream, or fresh parsley

1. Combine butternut squash, apples, onion, garlic, ginger, cinnamon, nutmeg, and turmeric in the slow cooker.

2. Add vegetable broth and stir to combine the ingredients.
Cover and cook on low for 4-6 hours or high for 2-3 hours, until the squash and apples are tender.

3. After cooking, use an immersion blender to puree the soup in the slow cooker. Alternatively, transfer the mixture to a blender in batches and process until smooth before returning it to the slow cooker.

4. Mix in coconut milk, lemon juice, and sea salt. Taste and adjust seasonings as necessary.

5. To serve, ladle the bisque into bowls and garnish with pumpkin seeds, coconut cream, or fresh parsley, as desired.

Tuscan White Bean & Kale Soup

Serves 6 Prep Time: 15 minutes Cooking Time: 6-8 hours (low) or 3-4 hours (high)

1 cup dried cannellini beans or 2 cans, drained and rinsed
6 cups vegetable broth (low-sodium)
1 medium onion, finely chopped
2 medium carrots, diced
3 celery stalks, diced
4 cloves garlic, minced
1 can (14 oz) diced tomatoes (no salt added)
2 cups fresh kale, chopped (stems removed)
1 teaspoon dried oregano
1 teaspoon dried thyme
1 teaspoon smoked paprika
1/2 teaspoon turmeric powder
1/4 teaspoon crushed red pepper flakes
1/4 teaspoon sea salt
1/4 teaspoon black pepper
1 tablespoon olive oil

1. For dried beans, rinse and soak overnight. Drain and rinse before putting in the slow cooker.

2. Add ingredients to the slow cooker. In a slow cooker, combine the dried beans, vegetable broth, onion, carrots, celery, garlic, diced tomatoes, oregano, thyme, smoked paprika, turmeric powder, and crushed red pepper flakes (if using). Stir to combine.

3. Cover and cook on low for 6-8 hours or high for 3-4 hours. If you use canned beans, add them in the last hour of cooking to avoid overcooking.

4. Stir in chopped kale in the last 30 minutes of cooking. Allow it to wilt and soften in the hot soup.

5. Taste and adjust seasoning with salt and pepper as needed.
Ladle the soup into bowls and drizzle with olive oil for extra flavor. Serve warm.

Red Lentil & Cauliflower Curry

Serves 4-6 Prep Time: 10 minutes Cooking Time: 4-6 hours (slow cooker)

1 cup red lentils, rinsed
1 small head cauliflower, cut into bite-sized florets
1 medium onion, diced
3 garlic cloves, minced
1 tablespoon fresh ginger, minced
1 tablespoon avocado oil
1 teaspoon ground turmeric
1 teaspoon ground cumin
1 teaspoon ground coriander
1/2 teaspoon paprika
1/4 teaspoon cayenne pepper
1 (14 oz) can unsweetened coconut milk
3 cups low-sodium vegetable broth or water
1 (14 oz) can diced tomatoes (no salt added)
1 cup baby spinach
1/2 teaspoon sea salt
Fresh cilantro
Fresh lime wedges

1. Sauté the Aromatics (Optional but recommended)
Warm the avocado oil in a skillet over medium heat.
Sauté the onion, garlic, and ginger for 2–3 minutes, until fragrant.
Add the turmeric, cumin, coriander, paprika, and cayenne (if using) and cook for another minute to toast the spices.

2. Assemble in the slow cooker. Transfer the sautéed mixture to a slow cooker. Combine the red lentils, cauliflower florets, diced tomatoes, coconut milk, and vegetable broth. Stir to combine.

3. Cover and cook on low for 6 hours or high for 4 hours, until the lentils and cauliflower are tender.

4. Stir spinach into the slow cooker for the last 10 minutes of cooking. The heat will wilt the leaves.

5. Taste the curry and adjust the seasoning with salt or lime juice.
Ladle the curry into bowls and top with fresh cilantro. Serve with lime wedges as a side.

Wild Rice & Mushroom Soup

Serves 6 Prep Time: 15 minutes Cooking Time: 6-8 hours (low) or 3-4 hours (high)

1 cup wild rice, rinsed
1 pound mixed mushrooms (e.g., cremini, shiitake, or oyster), sliced
2 celery stalks, diced
2 medium carrots, diced
1 medium onion, finely chopped
3 garlic cloves, minced
6 cups low-sodium vegetable broth
1 teaspoon turmeric powder
1 teaspoon dried thyme
1 teaspoon dried rosemary
1/2 teaspoon sea salt or to taste
1/4 teaspoon black pepper
1 cup raw cashews, soaked in water for 4-6 hours or boiled for 10 minutes
1 cup unsweetened almond milk or coconut milk
2 tablespoons fresh parsley, chopped

1. Prepare the slow cooker base. Place the wild rice, mushrooms, celery, carrots, onion, garlic, vegetable broth, turmeric, thyme, rosemary, sea salt, and black pepper (if using) in the slow cooker. Stir to combine.

2. Cover and cook on low for 6-8 hours or high for 3-4 hours until rice is tender and vegetables are soft.

3. Blend soaked cashews and almond milk until smooth and creamy.

4. Stir the cashew cream into the slow cooker 20 minutes before the soup finishes. Mix thoroughly and let the flavors meld together.

5. Ladle soup into bowls and garnish with fresh parsley before serving.

Mediterranean Quinoa Stew

Serves 6 Prep Time: 10 minutes Cooking Time: 4-6 hours on low or 2-3 hours on high

1 cup quinoa, rinsed and drained
2 cups vegetable broth (low-sodium or homemade)
1 can (14 oz) diced tomatoes (no salt added)
1 cup artichoke hearts, chopped (jarred in water, not oil)
1/2 cup pitted Kalamata olives, sliced
1 medium zucchini, diced
1 red bell pepper, diced
1 small onion, finely chopped
3 cloves garlic, minced

1 teaspoon dried oregano
1 teaspoon dried basil
1/2 teaspoon ground turmeric
1/4 teaspoon black pepper
1/4 teaspoon sea salt
1 tablespoon olive oil
2 tablespoons fresh parsley or cilantro, chopped

1. Rinse the quinoa thoroughly under cold water to remove any bitterness.
Chop all vegetables and herbs.

2. Add the rinsed quinoa, vegetable broth, diced tomatoes (including their juice), artichoke hearts, olives, zucchini, bell pepper, onion, garlic, oregano, basil, turmeric, black pepper (if using), and sea salt to the slow cooker. Stir to combine.

3. Cover the slow cooker and cook on low for 4-6 hours or high for 2-3 hours, until the quinoa is tender and the vegetables are cooked through.
Stir occasionally if possible, especially if cooking on high.

4. Spoon the stew into bowls and drizzle with olive oil. Garnish with fresh parsley or cilantro before serving.

Ginger-Garlic Bok Choy & Tofu Soup

Serves 4 Prep Time: 15 minutes Cooking Time: 4-6 hours on low or 2-3 hours on high

6 cups low-sodium vegetable broth
1 tablespoon fresh ginger, grated
3 cloves garlic, minced
1 tablespoon avocado oil or olive oil
2 medium carrots, thinly sliced
1 cup shiitake mushrooms, sliced or cremini mushrooms
1 block (14 ounces) extra-firm tofu, cubed
3 heads baby bok choy, halved lengthwise
2 tablespoons coconut aminos or low-sodium tamari
1 teaspoon turmeric powder
1/4 teaspoon black pepper
1/2 teaspoon sesame oil
2 green onions, thinly sliced
Fresh cilantro or parsley

1. Prepare the ingredients. In a small skillet, heat the avocado oil over medium heat. Sauté the ginger and garlic for 1-2 minutes, until fragrant.

2. Transfer the sautéed ginger and garlic to the slow cooker.
Pour in the vegetable broth and season with carrots, mushrooms, tofu, coconut aminos, turmeric, and black pepper (if using).

3. Cover and cook on low for 4-6 hours or high for 2-3 hours.
To avoid overcooking, add the bok choy to the slow cooker in the final 30 minutes.

4. Ladle soup into bowls. Drizzle with sesame oil and sprinkle with green onions, fresh cilantro, or parsley. Serve warm.

Silken Tofu with Bok Choy

Serves 4 Prep Time: 15 minutes Cooking Time: 4-5 hours on low or 2-3 hours on high

6 cups low-sodium vegetable broth
2 tablespoons white miso paste (added at the end)
1 tablespoon fresh ginger, grated
3 cloves garlic, minced
1 cup shiitake mushrooms, sliced
3 heads baby bok choy, halved lengthwise
1 block (14 ounces) silken tofu, cubed
2 teaspoons coconut aminos or low-sodium tamari
1 teaspoon turmeric powder
1/4 teaspoon black pepper
Juice of 1/2 lemon
Green onions, thinly sliced
Sesame seeds

1. In a slow cooker, combine vegetable broth, ginger, garlic, mushrooms, bok choy, and turmeric.

2. Gently place the cubed silken tofu in the slow cooker. Take care not to break it apart.

3. Cover and cook on low for 4-5 hours or high for 2-3 hours.

4. In the last 10 minutes of cooking, dissolve the miso paste in 1/4 cup warm water and stir it into the soup. Combine lemon juice and coconut aminos.

5. To serve, carefully ladle the soup into bowls.
Optional garnishes include green onions and sesame seeds. Serve warm.

Spiced Pumpkin & Split Pea Soup

Serves 6 Prep Time: 10 minutes Cooking Time: 6-8 hours (low) or 3-4 hours (high)

1 cup yellow split peas, rinsed and soaked for 1 hour
2 cups fresh pumpkin, peeled and diced or 1 can of pure pumpkin puree, unsweetened
1 small onion, finely chopped
2 cloves garlic, minced
1 teaspoon turmeric powder
1 teaspoon ground cumin
1/2 teaspoon ground coriander
1/2 teaspoon ground cinnamon
1/4 teaspoon cayenne pepper
1 teaspoon sea salt
1/4 teaspoon black pepper
4 cups vegetable broth (low sodium)
1 cup coconut milk (full fat, unsweetened)
1 tablespoon fresh ginger, grated
Juice of 1/2 lemon
fresh cilantro, toasted pumpkin seeds

1. Rinse and drain split peas after soaking.
If using fresh pumpkin, peel and cut it into small cubes.

2. Assemble in the slow cooker. Place the split peas, pumpkin, onion, garlic, turmeric, cumin, coriander, cinnamon, cayenne pepper (if using), sea salt, and black pepper in the slow cooker.
Pour in the vegetable broth and stir until combined.

3. Cover and cook on low for 6-8 hours or high for 3-4 hours, until split peas are tender and pumpkin is soft.

4. Once cooked, use an immersion blender to puree the soup to desired consistency. For a chunkier texture, blend half and leave the rest unblended. Stir in the coconut milk and grated ginger, and continue to warm the soup on low for 10 minutes.

5. Pour soup into bowls, top with lemon juice, cilantro, and toasted pumpkin seeds as desired.

Indian-Spiced Red Lentil & Spinach Dal

Serves 6 Prep Time: 10 minutes Cooking Time: 4-6 hours (on low)

1 cup red lentils, rinsed and drained
3 cups vegetable broth (low sodium)
1 cup full-fat coconut milk
3 cups fresh spinach, chopped
1 medium onion, finely diced
2 cloves garlic, minced
1-inch piece of fresh ginger, grated
1 teaspoon turmeric powder
1 teaspoon ground cumin
1 teaspoon ground coriander
1/2 teaspoon ground cinnamon
1/4 teaspoon cayenne pepper
1 teaspoon sea salt
Juice of 1 lemon
1 tablespoon coconut oil
Fresh cilantro, chopped

1. Rinse red lentils thoroughly and set aside. Chop the spinach, onion, and garlic; grate the ginger.

2. Assemble in a slow cooker. In a slow cooker, combine the red lentils, vegetable broth, coconut milk, onion, garlic, ginger, turmeric, cumin, coriander, cinnamon, and cayenne pepper (if using). Stir thoroughly to combine.

3. Cover and cook on low for 4-6 hours, or until the lentils are tender and creamy. Stir occasionally, if possible.

4. In the last 15 minutes of cooking, add chopped spinach and salt. Allow the spinach to wilt before incorporating into the dal.

5. After cooking, add lemon juice to enhance the flavors.

6. To serve, ladle the dal into bowls, garnish with fresh cilantro, and drizzle with melted coconut oil if desired. Serve alongside steamed basmati rice or gluten-free flatbread.

Barley & Root Vegetable Stew

Serves 6 Prep Time: 15 minutes Cooking Time: 6-8 hours on low or 3-4 hours on high

1 cup pearl barley, rinsed
2 medium carrots, peeled and diced
2 medium parsnips, peeled and diced
1 medium turnip, peeled and diced
1 medium onion, finely chopped
3 cloves garlic, minced
6 cups low-sodium vegetable broth
1 teaspoon turmeric powder
1 teaspoon dried thyme
1/2 teaspoon dried rosemary
1 bay leaf
1/2 teaspoon sea salt
1/4 teaspoon black pepper
2 cups chopped kale or spinach
1 tablespoon fresh parsley, chopped

1. Prepare the vegetables: Peel and dice carrots, parsnips, and turnips into bite-sized pieces. Chop the onions and mince the garlic.

2. Assemble the stew. Place the pearl barley, carrots, parsnips, turnips, onion, garlic, turmeric powder, thyme, rosemary, bay leaf, sea salt, and black pepper (if using) in the slow cooker.
Pour in the vegetable broth and stir until combined.

3. Cover the slow cooker and cook on **low** for 6-8 hours or **high** for 3-4 hours, until the barley and vegetables are tender.

4. Stir in chopped kale or spinach 20 minutes before serving. Let the greens wilt and soften.

5. To serve, remove the bay leaf and ladle the stew into bowls. Garnish with fresh parsley and serve warm.

Black Rice Porridge

Serves 4 Prep Time: 10 minutes Cooking Time: 4-6 hours (slow cooker)

1 cup black rice (also called forbidden rice), rinsed
4 cups water
1 cup unsweetened coconut milk (plus extra for drizzling)
1 tablespoon fresh ginger, finely grated
2 tablespoons dried goji berries or raisins, unsweetened

2 tablespoons maple syrup or raw honey
1/2 teaspoon ground cinnamon
1/4 teaspoon sea salt
toasted coconut flakes, chopped nuts (almonds or walnuts), fresh mango, or berries

1. Rinse black rice thoroughly with cold water until clear.

2. Combine the rinsed black rice, water, coconut milk, grated ginger, dried fruit, cinnamon, and sea salt in the slow cooker. Stir to combine.

3. Set the slow cooker to low and cook for 4-6 hours, stirring occasionally if possible. The rice should be tender, and the porridge creamy.
If the porridge becomes too thick while cooking, add more coconut milk or water until it reaches the desired consistency.

4. Add maple syrup or raw honey (if desired) just before serving.
Ladle the porridge into bowls and top with your favorite ingredients, such as fresh fruit, toasted coconut flakes, or chopped nuts. Drizzle with more coconut milk if desired.

Mexican-Style Pinto Bean Soup

Serves 6 Prep Time: 15 minutes Cooking Time: 6-8 hours (low) or 4-5 hours (high)

1 cup dried pinto beans, soaked overnight and rinsed or 3 cups cooked pinto beans
1 tablespoon avocado oil
1 small onion, diced
2 cloves garlic, minced
1 medium red bell pepper, diced
1 medium zucchini, diced
1 can (14.5 oz) fire-roasted diced tomatoes (no added salt)
4 cups low-sodium vegetable broth (or water)
1 cup fresh or frozen corn
1 teaspoon ground cumin
1 teaspoon smoked paprika
1/2 teaspoon ground coriander
1/2 teaspoon turmeric powder
1/4 teaspoon cayenne pepper
1/2 teaspoon sea salt
1/4 teaspoon black pepper
Juice of 1 lime
1/4 cup fresh cilantro, chopped
diced avocado, sliced jalapeños, lime wedges, or a dollop of coconut yogurt

1. Soak dried pinto beans overnight in water and thoroughly rinse before use. Dice all of the vegetables and gather the spices for easy assembly.

2. Heat avocado oil in a skillet over medium heat.
Sauté the onion, garlic, and red bell pepper for 3-4 minutes, until softened. This step improves flavor but can be skipped for convenience.

3. Assemble the soup. In a slow cooker, mix together the pinto beans, sautéed vegetables (if using), zucchini, fire-roasted tomatoes, corn, vegetable broth, and all spices. Stir to combine.

4. Cover and cook on low for 6-8 hours or high for 4-5 hours, until the beans are tender and the flavors combine.
- If you are using pre-cooked pinto beans, add them in the last hour of cooking to avoid overcooking.

5. To finish, add lime juice and cilantro just before serving.

6. To serve, ladle soup into bowls and top with desired toppings, such as diced avocado or coconut yogurt.

Creamy Cauliflower & White Bean Soup

Serves 6 Prep Time: 10 minutes Cooking Time: 4-6 hours (slow cooker)

1 medium head cauliflower, chopped into florets
1 can (15 oz) cannellini beans or great northern beans, rinsed and drained
1 medium onion, diced
3 garlic cloves, minced
4 cups low-sodium vegetable broth
1 teaspoon dried thyme
1/2 teaspoon turmeric powder
1/2 teaspoon ground cumin
1/2 teaspoon sea salt
1/4 teaspoon black pepper
1/2 cup canned coconut milk (full-fat or light)
1 tablespoon fresh lemon juice
2 tablespoons fresh parsley or chives, chopped

1. Cut cauliflower into small florets and dice onion. Rinse and drain the white beans.

2. Assemble the ingredients. Place the cauliflower, white beans, onion, garlic, vegetable broth, thyme, turmeric, cumin, sea salt, and black pepper (if using) in the slow cooker. Stir to combine.

3. Cover the slow cooker and cook on low for 6 hours or high for 4 hours until the cauliflower is tender.

4. Using an immersion blender, puree the soup in the slow cooker until creamy and smooth. Alternatively, transfer the soup to a blender in batches and puree until smooth (careful with hot liquids).

5. Stir in coconut milk and lemon juice to create a creamy and tangy finish. Taste and adjust the seasoning as needed.

6. Ladle soup into bowls and top with fresh parsley or chives. Serve warm.

Ethiopian-Style Red Lentil Stew

Serves 6 Prep Time: 15 minutes Cooking Time: 4-6 hours (low) or 2-3 hours (high)

1 tablespoon avocado oil or olive oil
1 medium onion, diced
3 garlic cloves, minced
1 tablespoon fresh ginger, grated
2 teaspoons berbere spice blend
1 teaspoon turmeric powder
1 1/2 cups red lentils, rinsed and drained
1 medium sweet potato, peeled and diced
1 can (14 oz) diced tomatoes, no salt added
4 cups low-sodium vegetable broth (or water)
1 bunch Swiss chard, stems removed and leaves chopped
1/2 teaspoon sea salt
Juice of 1 lemon
Chopped fresh cilantro
Lemon wedges

1. Heat avocado oil in a skillet over medium heat. Sauté the onion for 3-4 minutes, until softened. Cook for an additional 1-2 minutes, stirring in the garlic, ginger, berbere spice blend, and turmeric until fragrant.

2. Place the sautéed aromatics in the slow cooker. Combine the red lentils, sweet potato, diced tomatoes, and vegetable broth.

3. Cover and cook on low for 4-6 hours or high for 2-3 hours, until lentils and sweet potatoes are tender.

4. Stir in the chopped Swiss chard 15 minutes before the cooking time ends. Allow it to cook until wilted.

5. Add lemon juice to enhance the flavors. Adjust the salt as needed.

6. To serve, ladle the stew into bowls and garnish with fresh cilantro if desired. Serve lemon wedges on the side.

Mung Bean & Green Vegetable Soup

Serves 6 Prep Time: 15 minutes Cooking Time: 6-8 hours (low) or 3-4 hours (high)

1 cup dried mung beans, rinsed and soaked for 2-4 hours
1 medium onion, diced
2 garlic cloves, minced
1 tablespoon fresh ginger, grated
4 cups low-sodium vegetable broth
2 cups water
1 medium head of broccoli, cut into small florets
2 cups kale, chopped (stems removed)
1 medium zucchini, diced
1 teaspoon ground turmeric
1 teaspoon cumin powder
1/2 teaspoon black pepper
1/2 teaspoon sea salt
Juice of 1 lemon
2 tablespoons fresh cilantro, chopped

1. Soak mung beans for 2-4 hours to reduce cooking time and increase digestibility. Rinse thoroughly before using.

2. Assemble in a slow cooker. Place the soaked mung beans, onion, garlic, ginger, vegetable broth, water, turmeric, cumin, black pepper, and sea salt in the slow cooker. Stir to combine.

3. Cover and cook on low for 6-8 hours or high for 3-4 hours, until the mung beans tender.

4. Add the broccoli, kale, and zucchini (if using) to the slow cooker about 30 minutes before the soup is ready. Stir gently and cook until the vegetables are tender but vibrant.

5. Add lemon juice just before serving for a refreshing taste.
Ladle the soup into bowls and top with fresh cilantro, if desired.

Wild Rice & Cranberry Pilaf

Serves 6 Prep Time: 10 minutes Cooking Time: 4 hours on low or 2 hours on high

1 cup wild rice, rinsed
2 1/2 cups low-sodium vegetable broth
1/2 cup dried unsweetened cranberries
1/2 cup pecans, chopped (lightly toasted if desired)
1 small onion, finely diced
2 garlic cloves, minced
1 tablespoon avocado oil or olive oil
1 teaspoon dried thyme
1/2 teaspoon dried rosemary
1/4 teaspoon turmeric powder
1/4 teaspoon sea salt
1/4 teaspoon black pepper
2 tablespoons fresh parsley, chopped

1. Heat avocado oil in a skillet over medium heat. Saute the onion and garlic for 2-3 minutes, until softened.

2. Assemble in the slow cooker. Place the rinsed wild rice, vegetable broth, dried cranberries, pecans, sautéed onion and garlic, thyme, rosemary, turmeric, sea salt, and black pepper in the slow cooker. Stir thoroughly to combine.

3. Cover the slow cooker and cook on low for 4 hours or high for 2 hours until the rice is tender and the liquid has been absorbed.

4. Once cooked, use a fork to fluff the rice. Stir in the fresh parsley and adjust seasoning as needed.

5. Transfer to a serving dish and serve warm as a side dish or light main course.

8: SMOOTHIES, TEAS, AND BEVERAGES

Tart Cherry and Ginger Root

1 cup tart cherry juice (unsweetened)
1 inch fresh ginger root, peeled
1/2 cup frozen blueberries
1 tablespoon ground flaxseed
1/2 cup coconut water
1 small beet, peeled and chopped

Combine all ingredients in a blender
Blend until smooth

Golden Fennel Tea

1 fennel bulb, sliced
2 cardamom pods, crushed
1 teaspoon turmeric powder
1/4 teaspoon black pepper
2 cups water
1 tablespoon honey

1. Bring water to boil in a small pot
2. Add all ingredients except honey
3. Simmer for 15 minutes
4. Strain and add honey if desired

Inflammatory Power Fighter

1 cup purple cabbage, chopped
1 purple carrot
1 handful black grapes
1 tablespoon pomegranate seeds
1 cup coconut water
1/2 lemon, juiced
Small piece of fresh ginger

1. Juice all ingredients except coconut water
2. Mix with coconut water
3. Serve over ice

Rosemary-Sage Iced Tea

3 sprigs fresh rosemary
5 fresh sage leaves
2 cups boiling water
1 tablespoon raw honey
1/2 lemon, sliced
Ice cubes

1. Steep herbs in boiling water for 10 minutes
2. Strain and let cool
3. Add honey and lemon
4. Serve over ice

White Pine Needle and Blackberry Tea

2 tablespoons fresh white pine needles (from edible pine species only)
1/2 cup fresh blackberries
2 cups water
1 cinnamon stick
1 teaspoon raw honey

1. Bring water to a simmer
2. Add pine needles and cinnamon
3. Simmer for 20 minutes
4. Add crushed blackberries
5. Strain and sweeten if desired

Nettle and Mint Elixir

2 tablespoons dried nettle leaves
Fresh mint leaves
1 tablespoon apple cider vinegar
2 cups water
1 teaspoon raw honey
Pinch of sea salt

1. Steep nettle and mint in hot water for 15 minutes
2. Add apple cider vinegar and salt
3. Strain and sweeten with honey
4. Serve hot or cold

Celery-Cucumber Drink

3 celery stalks
1 cucumber
1 green apple
1 tablespoon fresh parsley
1/2 lime, juiced
1-inch piece of fresh turmeric
Pinch of black pepper

1. Juice all ingredients except lime and pepper
2. Add lime juice and pepper
3. Stir well and serve

Mushroom Latte

1 teaspoon reishi mushroom powder
1 teaspoon chaga mushroom powder
1 cup plant-based milk
1/2 teaspoon cinnamon
1/4 teaspoon vanilla extract
1 teaspoon MCT oil
Pinch of sea salt

1. Heat milk in a small pot
2. Whisk in all ingredients
3. Blend until frothy
4. Serve hot

Inflammation Relief Tea

1 tablespoon dried chamomile
1 tablespoon dried lemon balm
1 teaspoon dried rose petals
2 cups water
1/2 teaspoon vanilla extract
1 star anise pod

1. Bring water to boil
2. Add all ingredients
3. Steep for 10 minutes
4. Strain and serve

Bromelain Boost

1 cup fresh pineapple chunks
1/2 papaya, peeled and seeded
1 tablespoon fresh mint
1 thumb-sized piece of ginger
1/2 cup coconut water
1 tablespoon chia seeds
Ice cubes

1. Blend all ingredients until smooth
2. Add more coconut water if needed
3. Serve

9. LONG TERM MANAGEMENT ADVICE

So here we are, nearing the end of our journey together—or at least this portion of it. Before I let you go, let me share some of the most valuable lessons I've learned from my own anti-inflammatory journey.

First and foremost, figure out your triggers. Gluten, indoor mold, poor air quality, barometric pressure changes, and fragrances were all major concerns for me. It wasn't easy (or enjoyable) to figure it all out, but once I did, everything changed. And, yes, I've made some significant lifestyle changes—giving up gluten, investing in air purifiers, and scrutinizing every scented product as if I were auditioning for a fragrance-free detective show.

The truth is that determining environmental triggers is not always easy. Mold, for example, is a difficult one. There isn't a lot of solid research available, but believe me when mold makes you sick, you know. If you suspect something in your environment is to blame, try this simple test: avoid it for a few days before reintroducing yourself to it and seeing how you feel. Just don't bring anything porous (like clothes or furniture) that could harbor mold with you—trust me on this. It's like trying to leave a toxic relationship; you can't heal if you're still carrying parts of it with you.

Now, let us talk about food. When I first started, I had so many sensitivities that my diet felt like an ever-dwindling list of "no." However, working with a functional medicine doctor and addressing issues such as leaky gut (which is not a medical diagnosis but a functional issue that made a significant difference for me) allowed me to regain tolerance for many foods. Now I can enjoy a wide variety of yes foods, including leafy greens, colorful vegetables and fruits, healthy fats, and whole grains like quinoa and lentil pasta. Oh, and lots of garlic.

It is not only important to eat well, but also to live well. Get enough sleep, drink plenty of water, exercise regularly, and prioritize your mental health. Even your cookware is important—ditch the plastic and Teflon and invest in safer alternatives. Believe me, I've been down enough Google rabbit holes to know that even your frying pan can sabotage your health.

Anti-inflammatory superfoods like turmeric, cinnamon, and fresh herbs are more than just flavor enhancers; they are also life enhancers. Turmeric, in particular, is a powerhouse, but if you're supplementing, choose wisely. Some supplements are loaded with heavy metals or contain no active ingredients at all. Nobody likes a scam, especially when it is hidden in your health routine.

Here's the truth: there is no magic pill or one-size-fits-all solution for inflammation. The big picture includes your diet, sleep, exercise, mental health, and even the air you breathe. While this may sound overwhelming, it is also empowering. Because every small change you make takes you one step closer to feeling better, living better, and thriving in ways you never imagined.

So go ahead, start with one thing. Maybe it's incorporating more leafy greens into your meals. Perhaps it's replacing your old frying pan with a safer one. Perhaps it's time to get rid of that scented candle that gives you headaches every time you light it. Whatever it is, begin there. Then take the next step. And the next.

You've got it. You're on a journey, and there will be both challenges and setbacks, as well as breakthroughs and triumphs. And I will cheer you on from here, garlic breath and all.

4-Week Anti-Inflammatory Meal Plan

Week 1

Breakfast
- Monday: Scrambled Eggs with Sumac (p.15)
- Tuesday: Buckwheat and Chia Seed Porridge (p.18)
- Wednesday: Oat Porridge with Berries (p.19)
- Thursday: Breakfast Burritos with Refried Beans (p.20)
- Friday: Whole Grain Toast with Egg (p.23)
- Saturday: Avocado on Sprouted Grain Toast (p.26)
- Sunday: Blueberry Buckwheat Pancakes (p.28)

Lunch
- Monday: Sautéed Tomatoes and Mushrooms (p.31)
- Tuesday: Spinach and Chickpea Curry with Rice (p.56)
- Wednesday: Grilled Vegetable and Pesto Pasta (p.34)
- Thursday: Black Bean and Sweet Potato Tacos (p.35)
- Friday: Mushroom and Garlic Quinoa Salad (p.52)
- Saturday: Kale and Sweet Potato Salad (p.61)
- Sunday: Asian Slaw (p.58)

Dinner
- Monday: Thai Red Curry with Tofu over Rice (p.36)
- Tuesday: Chickpea and Lentil Curry (p.41)
- Wednesday: Wild Rice and Mushroom Soup (p.88)
- Thursday: Moroccan Chickpea and Quinoa Soup (p.83)
- Friday: Grilled Mackerel with Ginger (p.73)
- Saturday: Poached Salmon with Herbs (p.75)
- Sunday: Golden Lentil and Sweet Potato Stew (p.82)

Snacks/Drinks
- Tart Cherry and Ginger Root Drink (p.102)
- Celery-Cucumber Drink (p.108)
- Rosemary-Sage Iced Tea (p.105)

Week 2

Breakfast
- Monday: Tofu Scramble on Corn Tortilla with Salsa (p.17)
- Tuesday: Chia Pudding Topped with Goji Berries (p.24)
- Wednesday: Smoked Salmon, Avocado, and Poached Eggs (p.30)

- Thursday: Breakfast Burritos with Refried Beans (p.20)
- Friday: Sprouted Grain English Muffins (p.25)
- Saturday: Avocado Toast with Sriracha (p.27)
- Sunday: Blueberry, Banana, and Muffins (p.22)

Lunch
- Monday: Couscous with Chickpea Stew (p.38)
- Tuesday: Mediterranean Hummus Collard Wrap (p.70)
- Wednesday: Chickpea Rice Pasta Primavera (p.50)
- Thursday: Lettuce Wraps with Smoked Trout (p.63)
- Friday: Teff and Vegetable Pilaf (p.44)
- Saturday: Quinoa Vegetable Wrap (p.65)
- Sunday: Rainbow Lettuce Boats (p.69)

Dinner
- Monday: Herb-Crusted Halibut with Mashed Cauliflower (p.80)
- Tuesday: Tuscan White Bean and Kale Soup (p.86)
- Wednesday: Spaghetti Squash with Asparagus (p.54)
- Thursday: Ethiopian-Style Red Lentil Stew (p.98)
- Friday: Red Lentil and Cauliflower Curry (p.87)
- Saturday: Indian-Spiced Red Lentil and Spinach Dal (p.93)
- Sunday: Mediterranean Quinoa Stew (p.89)

Snacks/Drinks
- Inflammation Relief Tea (p.110)
- Bromelain Boost (p.111)
- Mushroom Latte (p.109)

Week 3

Breakfast
- Monday: Oat Porridge with Berries (p.19)
- Tuesday: Scrambled Eggs with Dill (p.29)
- Wednesday: Tofu Shakshuka (p.16)
- Thursday: Buckwheat and Chia Seed Porridge (p.18)
- Friday: Avocado on Sprouted Grain Toast (p.26)
- Saturday: Blueberry Buckwheat Pancakes (p.28)
- Sunday: Smoked Salmon, Avocado, and Poached Eggs (p.30)

Lunch
- Monday: Farro Risotto with Butternut Squash (p.53)
- Tuesday: Black Rice Asian Bowl (p.47)
- Wednesday: Asian-Inspired Rice Paper Rolls (p.66)
- Thursday: Greek Chickpea Salad (p.60)
- Friday: Chickpea Egg Salad Wrap (p.64)
- Saturday: Mexican Black Bean Lettuce Wraps (p.67)

- Sunday: Kale and Sweet Potato Salad (p.61)

Dinner
- Monday: Barley and Root Vegetable Stew (p.94)
- Tuesday: Wild Rice and Cranberry Pilaf (p.100)
- Wednesday: Butternut Squash and Apple Bisque (p.85)
- Thursday: Spaghetti Squash Garlic Noodles (p.55)
- Friday: Moroccan Chickpea and Quinoa Soup (p.83)
- Saturday: Halloumi Peanut Curry (p.39)
- Sunday: Mung Bean and Green Vegetable Soup (p.99)

Snacks/Drinks
- Nettle and Mint Elixir (p.107)
- Golden Fennel Tea (p.103)
- Celery-Cucumber Drink (p.108)

Week 4

Breakfast
- Monday: Avocado Toast with Sriracha (p.27)
- Tuesday: Chia Pudding Topped with Goji Berries (p.24)
- Wednesday: Blueberry, Banana, and Muffins (p.22)
- Thursday: Sprouted Grain English Muffins (p.25)
- Friday: Whole Grain Toast with Egg (p.23)
- Saturday: Oat Porridge with Berries (p.19)
- Sunday: Breakfast Burritos with Refried Beans (p.20)

Lunch
- Monday: Red Rice Mexican Bowl (p.45)
- Tuesday: Lentil and Brown Rice Pilaf (p.51)
- Wednesday: Mediterranean Hummus Collard Wrap (p.70)
- Thursday: Chickpea and Vegetable Frittata (p.42)
- Friday: Asian Slaw (p.58)
- Saturday: Quinoa and Citrus Salad (p.71)
- Sunday: Chickpea Rice Pasta Primavera (p.50)

Dinner
- Monday: Wild Rice and Mushroom Soup (p.88)
- Tuesday: Tuscan White Bean and Kale Soup (p.86)
- Wednesday: Indian-Spiced Red Lentil and Spinach Dal (p.93)
- Thursday: Chickpea and Lentil Curry (p.41)
- Friday: Garlic and Chili Veggie Stir-Fry Noodles (p.37)
- Saturday: Thai Red Curry with Tofu over Rice (p.36)
- Sunday: Herb-Crusted Halibut with Mashed Cauliflower (p.80)

Snacks/Drinks

- Tart Cherry and Ginger Root Drink (p.102)
- White Pine Needle and Blackberry Tea (p.106)
- Mushroom Latte (p.109)

Recipe Index

A
Amaranth Porridge Bowl (p.46)
Asian-Inspired Rice Paper Rolls (p.66)
Asian Slaw (p.58)
Avocado on Sprouted Grain Toast (p.26)
Avocado Toast with Sriracha (p.27)

B
Baked Cod with Mediterranean Flavors (p.74)
Barley and Root Vegetable Stew (p.94)
Berry Almond Butter Wrap (p.68)
Black Bean and Sweet Potato Tacos (p.35)
Black Rice Asian Bowl (p.47)
Black Rice Porridge (p.95)
Blueberry, Banana, and Muffins (p.22)
Blueberry Buckwheat Pancakes (p.28)
Bromelain Boost (p.111)
Buckwheat and Chia Seed Porridge (p.18)
Butternut Squash and Apple Bisque (p.85)

C
Celery-Cucumber Drink (p.108)
Chia Pudding Topped with Goji Berries (p.24)
Chickpea Curry (p.41)
Chickpea Egg Salad Wrap (p.64)
Chickpea Mayo (p.40)
Chickpea Rice Pasta Primavera (p.50)
Chickpea Tuna Salad Sandwich (p.76)
Couscous with Chickpea Stew (p.38)
Creamy Cauliflower and White Bean Soup (p.97)

E
Ethiopian-Style Red Lentil Stew (p.98)

F
Farro Risotto with Butternut Squash (p.53)

G
Garlic and Chili Veggie Stir-Fry Noodles (p.37)
Golden Fennel Tea (p.103)
Golden Lentil and Sweet Potato Stew (p.82)

Grilled Mackerel with Ginger (p.73)
Grilled Vegetable and Pesto Pasta (p.34)

H
Halloumi Peanut Curry (p.39)
Herb-Crusted Halibut with Mashed Cauliflower (p.80)

I
Indian-Spiced Red Lentil and Spinach Dal (p.93)
Inflammation Relief Tea (p.110)

K
Kale and Sweet Potato Salad (p.61)
King Oyster Mushroom Scallops (p.77)

L
Lentil and Brown Rice Pilaf (p.51)
Lentil Tabbouleh (p.62)
Lettuce Wraps with Smoked Trout (p.63)

M
Mediterranean Hummus Collard Wrap (p.70)
Mexican Black Bean Lettuce Wraps (p.67)
Mexican-Style Pinto Bean Soup (p.96)
Millet Mediterranean Bowl (p.48)
Moroccan Chickpea and Quinoa Soup (p.83)
Mung Bean and Green Vegetable Soup (p.99)
Mushroom and Garlic Quinoa Salad (p.52)
Mushroom and Brown Rice Congee (p.84)
Mushroom Latte (p.109)

N
Nettle and Mint Elixir (p.107)

O
Oat Porridge with Berries (p.19)

P
Plant-Based Vegetable Frittata (p.42)
Poached Salmon with Herbs (p.75)

Q
Quinoa and Citrus Salad (p.71)
Quinoa Vegetable Wrap (p.65)

R
Rainbow Lettuce Boats (p.69)

Red Lentil and Cauliflower Curry (p.87)
Red Rice Mexican Bowl (p.45)
Rosemary-Sage Iced Tea (p.105)

S
Sautéed Tomatoes and Mushrooms (p.31)
Scrambled Eggs with Dill (p.29)
Scrambled Eggs with Sumac (p.15)
Sheet Pan Cauliflower Tacos (p.21)
Silken Tofu with Bok Choy (p.91)
Smoked Salmon, Avocado, and Poached Eggs (p.30)
Spaghetti Squash Garlic Noodles (p.55)
Spaghetti Squash with Asparagus (p.54)
Spiced Pumpkin and Split Pea Soup (p.92)
Spinach and Chickpea Curry with Rice (p.56)
Sprouted Grain English Muffins (p.25)
Stir-Fried Tofu and Vegetables (p.33)

T
Tart Cherry and Ginger Root Drink (p.102)
Teff and Vegetable Pilaf (p.44)
Tempeh Fish Fillets (p.79)
Thai Red Curry with Tofu over Rice (p.36)
Tofu Crab Cakes (p.78)
Tofu Scramble on Corn Tortilla with Salsa (p.17)
Tofu Shakshuka (p.16)
Tuscan White Bean and Kale Soup (p.86)

W
Wild Rice and Cranberry Pilaf (p.100)
Wild Rice and Mushroom Bowl (p.49)
Wild Rice and Mushroom Soup (p.88)
Whole Grain Toast with Egg (p.23)

Y
White Pine Needle and Blackberry Tea (p.106)

Printed in Great Britain
by Amazon